EIGHTH EDITION

Bontrager's
HANDBOOK OF
RADIOGRAPHIC
POSITIONING
AND **TECHNIQUES**

Kenneth L. Bontrager, MA

John P. Lampignano, MEd, RT(R)(CT)

ELSEVIER
MOSBY

3251 Riverport Lane
St. Louis, Missouri 63043

BONTRAGER'S HANDBOOK OF RADIOGRAPHIC   ISBN: 978-0-323-08389-8
POSITIONING AND TECHNIQUES, EIGHTH EDITION

Notices

Knowledge and best practice in this field are constantly changing. As new research
and experience broaden our understanding, changes in research methods,
professional practices, or medical treatment may become necessary.

Practitioners and researchers must always rely on their own experience and
knowledge in evaluating and using any information, methods, compounds, or
experiments described herein. In using such information or methods they should be
mindful of their own safety and the safety of others, including parties for whom
they have a professional responsibility.

With respect to any drug or pharmaceutical products identified, readers are
advised to check the most current information provided (i) on procedures featured
or (ii) by the manufacturer of each product to be administered, to verify the
recommended dose or formula, the method and duration of administration, and
contraindications. It is the responsibility of practitioners, relying on their own
experience and knowledge of their patients, to make diagnoses, to determine
dosages and the best treatment for each individual patient, and to take all
appropriate safety precautions.

To the fullest extent of the law, neither the Publisher nor the authors,
contributors, or editors, assume any liability for any injury and/or damage to
persons or property as a matter of products liability, negligence or otherwise,
or from any use or operation of any methods, products, instructions, or ideas
contained in the material herein.

ISBN: 978-0-323-08389-8

Executive Content Strategist: Jennifer Janson
Content Development Specialist: Amy Whittier
Publishing Services Manager: Catherine Jackson
Senior Production Editor: Carol O'Connell

Printed in United States of America

Last digit is the print number:
9 8 7 6 5 4 3 2

Preface

This pocket handbook was first developed by Ken Bontrager in 1994 as a response to the need by students and technologists alike for a more thorough and still practical pocket guide covering the applied aspects of radiographic positioning and techniques (exposure factors). Today this compact and durable pocket-sized handbook still includes a review of all the common imaging procedures, yet is small enough to be easily carried in clinical situations. Sufficient space is included for writing personal notes and exposure techniques that technologists find work for them with specific equipment, or in certain rooms or departments.

Positioning descriptions and photographs are provided for each projection/position, along with CR locations, degrees of obliquity, specific CR angles, AEC cell locations, patient shielding, and suggested kV ranges. A quick review of this information before beginning a procedure can provide assurance that the exam is being correctly performed with the least possible patient dose.

Standard Radiographic Image and Evaluation Criteria

The eighth edition of this handbook includes a standard, well-positioned radiograph with each position described. Also added with these standard radiographic images is a brief summary of quality factors to be used as a critique guide. Viewing this radiograph and comparing it with the list of evaluation criteria leads users through a critique of the image they are viewing or have just taken by comparing it to that of this standard.

Also included is an optional competency sign-off check to be signed by the clinical instructor for individual student competency records if so desired.

Acknowledgments

Jennifer Janson, Amy Whittier, and Carol O'Connell from Elsevier Publishing were instrumental in providing support, guidance, and the resources in the redesign and publishing of the pocket handbook. We are most indebted to our former students, fellow technologists, and those many educators throughout the United States and Canada who challenged and inspired us. We thank all of you and hope this pocket handbook continues to be a valuable aid in improving and maintaining that high level of radiographic imaging for which we all strive.

Acknowledgments

Contents

Contents

Explanations for Use

This handbook is intended as a quick reference and review and assumes that each user has successfully completed, or is now completing, courses in radiographic positioning and procedures.

Radiation protection: Certain radiation protection practices and shielding descriptions are included with each projection and **it is the responsibility of the technologist to ensure that maximum shielding is used wherever possible.**

Patient doses: Methods to reduce effective dose including collimation, shielding, and technical considerations given for each projection. (See Appendix A for more details.)

kV ranges: Suggested kV ranges for analog and digital systems are **stated** for each projection. These are estimates based on common practice from several facilities and validated by imaging experts. **These kV ranges may not apply to every department protocol or imaging systems employed.** The technologist should consult with their radiation safety officer or supervisor to determine appropriate kV ranges for their clinical setting.

Chapter title pages: The list of projections with page numbers is at the beginning of each chapter for ease in locating specific projections and also as a reference for marking the basic department routines for each examination. A small check √ can be placed in the box by each projection that is part of the preferred departmental routine. Each projection is also followed with either an **(R)** or a **(S)** for a suggested departmental **routine** or **special.**

Standard Radiographic Image and Evaluation Criteria: With each positioning page is a **standard radiograph** of that projection. Viewing this radiograph and comparing it with the list of **evaluation criteria** to check leads the user through a critique of the image they are reviewing by comparing it to the standard radiograph.

Also included is an optional **competency sign-off area** to be signed by the clinical instructor for individual student competency records.

Each positioning page has a format similar to this sample page.

1. Suggested location of patient ID info. For chest exams this represents the top right of the image receptor (IR).

2. Recommended AEC chamber(s) (darkened R and L upper cells indicated on this PA chest example). **Note:** Verify AEC chamber selection with department before employing.

3. Collimation field size with CR location in center.

4. IR size recommended for average adult, placed lengthwise (L.W.) for portrait, or crosswise (C.W.) for landscape in reference to the patient. Grid or nongrid.

5. Patient position description.

6. CR location and CR angle.

7. Suggested SID range.

8. Suggested kV ranges. Analog and digital systems. (Pencil in kV range for your imaging systems.)

9. Imaging factors to be filled in (in pencil) as determined best for small (S), medium (M), or large (L) patients, or for specific rooms.

10. This additional space is provided for exposure factors for analog systems or for specific types of digital image receptors that require technique adjustments.

11. Corresponding page number in textbook for projection.

PA Chest

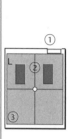

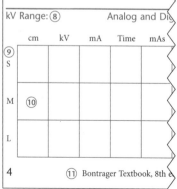

①

L ②

③

- 35 × 43 cm L.W. or C.W. (14 × 17″) ④
- Grid

Fig. 1-2 P below ver female, 18 ⌀

Position ⑤
- Erect, chin raised, hands on hips with pa forward
- Center CR to T7 region. Top of IR will b above shoulders on **average** patient.
- Center thorax bilaterally to IR borders w sides; ensure there is **no rotation** of tho

Central Ray: CR ⊥, to T7, or 7-8″ (18-20 ⑥ prominens (is also near level of inferior

SID: 72-120″ (183 to 307 cm) ⑦

Collimation: Upper border to vertebra pr skin borders

Respiration: Expose at end of **2nd deep in**

kV Range: ⑧　　　　　　Analog and Di

	cm	kV	mA	Time	mAs
⑨ S					
M ⑩					
L					

4　　　　⑪ Bontrager Textbook, 8th e

Explanations for Use

vii

Chapter 1

Chest

(R) Routine, (S) Special

Chest

1

1

Chest—Positioning Considerations and Radiation Protection

Collimation

Restricting the primary beam coverage is a very effective way to reduce patient exposure in chest radiography. This requires accurate and correct location of the central ray (CR).

Correct CR Location

Correct CR location to the midchest (T7) allows for accurate collimation and protection of the upper radiosensitive region of the neck area. It also prevents exposure to the dense abdominal area below the diaphragm, which produces scatter and secondary radiation to the radiosensitive reproductive organs.

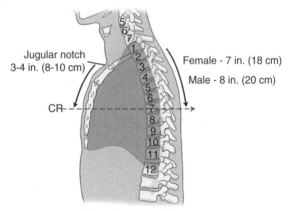

Jugular notch
3-4 in. (8-10 cm)

Female - 7 in. (18 cm)
Male - 8 in. (20 cm)

CR

Fig. 1-1 Correct CR location.

T7 for the **PA chest** can be located posteriorly in reference to C7, the **vertebra prominens.** Level of T7 is 7-8 inches (18-20 cm) below the vertebra prominens.

The CR for the **AP chest** is 3-4 inches (8-11 cm) below the **jugular notch** and angled 3°-5° caudad.

Bontrager Textbook, 8th ed, pp. 83 and 84.

Shielding

Shielding of radiosensitive organs and tissues should be used for all procedures unless it obscures key anatomy. Shielding is not a substitute for close collimation.

Backscatter Protection

Shields placed between the patient and the wall Bucky and wall can also be used to keep scatter and secondary radiation from these structures from reaching the patient's gonadal regions.

Digital Imaging Considerations

The following technical factors will reduce dose to the patient and improve image quality:

Collimation: Close collimation reduces dose to the patient and scatter radiation reaching the image receptor.

Accurate Centering: Most digital systems recommend that the anatomy be centered to the receptor.

kV Range: Digital systems allow the use of higher kV as compared to analog (film-based) systems, which will reduce patient dose.

Exposure Indicator: Check the exposure indicator to verify that the optimal exposure factors were used to produce the least amount of radiation to the patient.

Grids: Grids generally are not used with analog (film-screen) imaging for body parts measuring 10 cm or less. However, with certain digital systems, the grid may or may not be able to be removed from the receptor. In those cases it is departmental protocol that determines if a grid is left in place or removed.

PA Chest

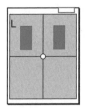

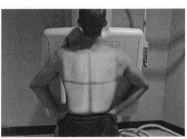

- 35 × 43 cm L.W. or C.W. (14 × 17")
- Grid

Fig. 1-2 PA chest (CR ≈20 cm [8"] below vertebra prominens) (average female, 18 cm [7"]).

Position

- Erect, chin raised, hands on hips with palms out, roll shoulders forward
- Center CR to T7 region. Top of IR will be approximately 2" (5 cm) above shoulders on **average** patient.
- Center thorax bilaterally to IR borders with equal margins on both sides; ensure there is **no rotation** of thorax.

Central Ray: CR ⊥, to T7, or 7-8" (18-20 cm) below vertebra prominens (is also near level of inferior angle of scapula)

SID: 72-120" (183 to 307 cm)

Collimation: Upper border to vertebra prominens; sides to lateral skin borders

Respiration: Expose at end of **2nd deep inspiration.**

---

kV Range:			Analog and Digital Systems: **110-125 kV**			
	cm	kV	mA	Time	mAs	SID	Exposure Indicator
S							
M							
L							

Bontrager Textbook, 8th ed, p. 90.

Lateral Chest

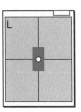

- 35 × 43 cm L.W. (14 × 17″)
- Grid

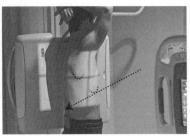

Fig. 1-3 Left lateral chest.

Chest

Position

- Erect, left side against IR (unless right lateral is indicated)
- Arms raised, crossed above head, chin up
- **True lateral,** no rotation or tilt. Midsagittal plane parallel to IR (Don't push hips in against the IR holder.)
- Thorax centered to CR, and to IR anteriorly and posteriorly

Central Ray: CR ⊥, to midthorax at level of T7. Generally IR and CR should be lowered ≈1″ (2.5 cm) from PA on average patient.

SID: 72-120″ (183-307 cm)

Collimation: Upper border to level of vertebra prominens, sides to anterior and posterior skin margins

Respiration: Expose at end of **2nd full inspiration.**

kV Range:			Analog and Digital Systems: 110-125 kV				
	cm	kV	mA	Time	mAs	SID	Exposure Indicator
S							
M							
L							

Lateral, Wheelchair or Stretcher

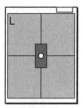

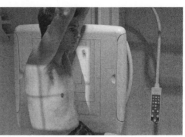

Fig. 1-4 Left lateral on stretcher.

- 35 × 43 cm L.W. (14 × 17″)
- Grid

Position
- Erect, on stretcher or in wheelchair
- Arms raised, crossed above head, or hold on to support bar
- Center thorax to CR, and to IR anteriorly and posteriorly
- No rotation or tilt, midsagittal plane parallel to IR, keep chin up

Central Ray: CR ⊥, to midthorax at level of T7

SID: 72-120″ (183-307 cm)

Collimation: Upper border to level of vertebra prominens, sides to anterior and posterior skin margins

Respiration: Expose at end of **2nd full inspiration.**

kV Range:			Analog and Digital Systems: 110-125 kV			
	cm	kV	mA	Time	mAs	SID	Exposure Indicator
S							
M							
L							

Bontrager Textbook, 8th ed, p. 93.

PA (AP) Chest

Evaluation Criteria
Anatomy Demonstrated:
- Both lungs from apices to costophrenic angles
- 9-10 ribs demonstrated above the diaphragm

Position:
- Chin sufficiently elevated
- No rotation, SC joints and lateral rib margins equal distance from spine

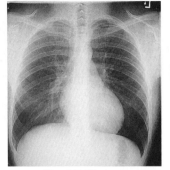

Fig. 1-5 PA chest.

Competency Check: _____

Technologist   Date

Exposure:
- No motion, sharp outlines of diaphragm and lung markings visible
- Exposure sufficient to visualize faint outlines of midthoracic and upper thoracic vertebrae through heart and mediastinal structures

---

Lateral Chest

Evaluation Criteria
Anatomy Demonstrated:
- From apices to costophrenic angles, from sternum to posterior ribs

Position:
- Chin and arms elevated to prevent superimposing apices
- No rotation, R and L posterior ribs superimposed except side away from IR projected slightly (1-2 cm) posteriorly because of divergent rays

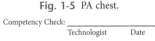

Fig. 1-6 Lateral chest.

Competency Check: _____

Technologist   Date

Exposure:
- No motion, sharp outlines of diaphragm and lung markings
- Sufficient exposure and contrast to visualize rib outlines and lung markings through heart shadow

Lateral Decubitus

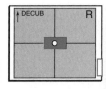

- 35 × 43 cm (14 × 17″) L.W. with respect to patient
- Grid

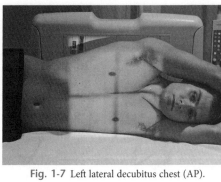

Fig. 1-7 Left lateral decubitus chest (AP).

Position
- Patient on side (R or L, see *Note*) with pad under patient
- Ensure that stretcher does not move (lock wheels)
- Raise both arms above head, chin up
- True AP, no rotation, patient centered to CR at level of T7

Central Ray: CR horizontal to T7, 3-4″ (8-10 cm) below jugular notch

SID: 72-120″ (183-307 cm) with wall Bucky; 40-44″ (102-113 cm) with erect table and Bucky

Collimation: Collimate on four sides to area of lung fields (top border of light field to level of vertebra prominens).

Respiration: End of **2nd full inspiration**

Note: For possible fluid (pleural effusion), suspected side down; possible air (pneumothorax), suspected side up.

---

kV Range: Analog and Digital Systems: 110-125 kV

	cm	kV	mA	Time	mAs	SID	Exposure Indicator
S							
M							
L							

Bontrager Textbook, 8th ed, p. 95.

AP Lordotic

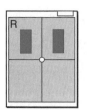

- 35 × 43 cm L.W. (14 × 17″)
- Grid

Position

- Patient stands ≈1 ft (30 cm) away from IR, leans back against chest board
- Hands on hips, palms out, shoulders rolled forward
- Center midsternum and IR to CR, top of **IR** should be 3-4″ (8-10 cm) above shoulders

Central Ray: CR⊥to IR, 10-12 cm below jugular notch

SID: 72-120″ (183-307 cm)

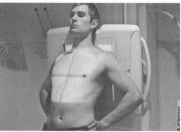

Fig. 1-8 AP lordotic (best demonstrates apices of lungs).

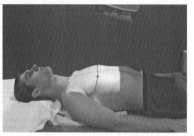

Fig. 1-9 AP supine, CR 15-20″ cephalad.

Chest

Collimation: Collimate on four sides to area of lung fields (top border of light field to level of vertebra prominens).

Respiration: End of **2nd full inspiration**

	cm	kV	mA	Time	mAs	SID	Exposure Indicator
kV Range:		Analog and Digital Systems: 110-125 kV					
S							
M							
L							

Lateral Decubitus Chest—AP (PA)

Evaluation Criteria
Anatomy Demonstrated:
- Entire lung fields, including apices and costophrenic angles

Position:
- No rotation, equal distance from lateral rib borders to spine

Exposure:
- No motion; diaphragm, ribs, and lung markings appear sharp

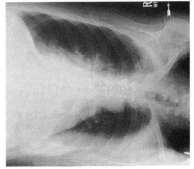

Fig. 1-10 Left lateral decubitus.

Competency Check: _____
Technologist   Date

- Faint visualization of vertebrae and ribs through heart shadow

---

AP Lordotic Chest

Evaluation Criteria
Anatomy Demonstrated:
- Entire lung fields; include clavicles, which should appear above apices

Position:
- Clavicles appear nearly horizontal, superior to apices
- No rotation as evident by equal distance between medial ends of clavicles and lateral borders of ribs and spinal column

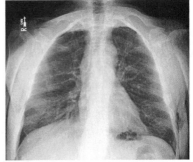

Fig. 1-11 AP lordotic chest.

Competency Check: _____
Technologist   Date

Exposure:
- No motion; diaphragm, heart, and rib borders appear sharp
- Optimum contrast and density (brightness and contrast for digital images) to visualize vertebral outlines through mediastinal structures

Anterior Oblique Chest (RAO and LAO)

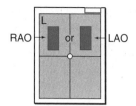

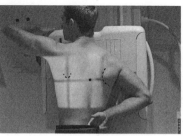

Fig. 1-12 45° RAO.

- 35 × 43 cm L.W.
  (14 × 17″)
- Grid

Position

- Erect, rotated 45°, right shoulder against IR holder (RAO)
  (Certain heart studies require LAO, 60° rotation from PA.)
- Arm away from IR up resting on head or on IR holder
- Arm nearest IR down on hip, keep chin up
- Center thorax laterally to IR margins; vertically to CR at T7

Central Ray: CR ⊥, to level of T7

SID: 72-120″ (183-307 cm)

Collimation: Collimate on four sides to area of lung fields (top
border of light field to level of vertebra prominens).

Respiration: End of **2nd full inspiration**

Note: Site of interest should be farthest from IR on anterior oblique,
and closest to IR on posterior oblique.

kV Range:			Analog and Digital Systems: 110-125 kV				
	cm	kV	mA	Time	mAs	SID	Exposure Indicator
S							
M							
L							

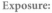

Evaluation Criteria

Anatomy Demonstrated:

- Included both lung fields from apices to costophrenic angles

Position:

- With 45° rotation, distance from outer rib borders to vertebral column on side farthest from IR should be approximately 2 times distance of side closest to IR.

Exposure:

- No motion; diaphragm and rib margins appear sharp
- Vascular markings throughout lungs and rib outlines visualized faintly through heart

Notes:

- Anterior oblique projections best demonstrate the side farthest from IR.
- Less rotation (15-20° may better visualize areas of lungs for possible pulmonary disease)
- Posterior oblique projections best visualize side closest to IR.

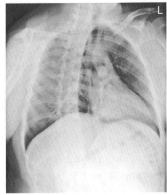

Fig 1-13 45° RAO.

Competency Check: _____
Technologist   Date

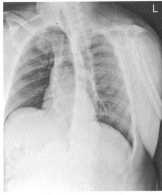

Fig. 1-14 45° LAO.

Competency Check: _____
Technologist   Date

AP and Lateral Upper Airway
(Trachea and Larynx)

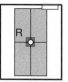

- 24 × 30 cm L.W. (10 × 12″)
- Grid

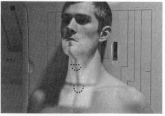

Fig. 1-15 AP.

Position
- Erect, seated or standing, center upper airway to CR
- Arms down, chin raised slightly
- Lateral: Depress shoulders and pull shoulders back
- Center of IR to level of CR

Central Ray: CR ⊥, to midpoint between lower margin of thyroid cartilage and jugular notch (C6–C7);

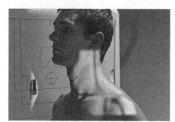

Fig. 1-16 Lateral.

or ≈2″ (5 cm) lower if trachea is of primary interest

SID: 72-120″ (183-307 cm)

Collimation: Collimate to region of soft tissue neck.

Respiration: Expose during slow, gentle inspiration.

kV Range:			Analog and Digital Systems: 75-85 kV			
	cm	kV	mA	Time	mAs	SID	Exposure Indicator
S							
M							
L							

Chest

AP and Lateral Upper Airway

Evaluation Criteria
Anatomy Demonstrated:
AP and Lateral
- Larynx and trachea well visualized, filled with air

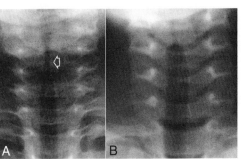

Fig. 1-17 AP upper airway.

Competency Check: _____
Technologist   Date

Position:
AP
- No rotation, symmetric appearance of sternoclavicular joints
- Mandible superimposes base of skull

Lateral
- To visualize neck region, include EAM at upper border of image.
- If distal larynx and trachea is of primary interest, center lower to include area from C3 to T5 (Fig. 1-18).

Exposure:
AP
- Optimum exposure visualizes air-filled trachea through C and T vertebrae.

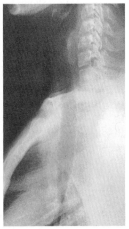

Fig. 1-18 Lateral upper airway.

Competency Check: _____
Technologist Date

Lateral
- Optimum exposure includes air-filled larynx, and upper trachea not overexposed
- Cervical and thoracic vertebrae will appear underexposed.

14

AP Pediatric Chest

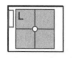

- 18 × 24 cm or 24 × 30 cm C.W. (8 × 10″ or 10 × 12″)
- TT (tabletop; nongrid). Grid with systems when it can't be removed.

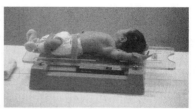

Fig. 1-19 Immobilization device.

Chest

Position

- Supine, arms and legs extended, tape and sandbags or other immobilization of arms and legs
- No rotation of thorax, gonadal shield over pelvic area
- IR and thorax centered to CR

Central Ray: CR ⊥, to midlung fields, mammillary (nipple) line

SID: Minimum 50-60″ (128-153 cm); x-ray tube raised as high as possible

Collimation: Closely collimate on four sides to outer chest margins.

Respiration: Full inspiration; if crying, time the exposure at full inhalation

Note: If parental assistance is necessary, have parent hold arms overhead with head tilted back with one hand, and other hand holding down legs (provide with lead apron and gloves).

	cm	kV	mA	Time	mAs	SID	Exposure Indicator
S							
M							
L							

kV Range: Analog: 70-80 kV   Digital Systems: 75-85 kV

Bontrager Textbook, 8th ed, p. 631.   15

Erect PA Pediatric Chest (with Pigg-O-Stat)

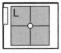

- 18 × 24 cm or 24 × 30 cm C.W. (8 × 10″ or 10 × 12″)
- IR (nongrid) or grid with systems when it can't be removed

Chest

Position

- Patient on seat, legs through openings
- Adjust height of seat to place shoulders ≈1″ (2.5 cm) below upper margin of IR.

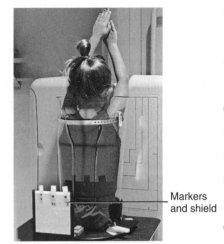

Markers and shield

Fig. 1-20 PA chest (Pigg-O-Stat, for 5-year-old) (DR)

- Raise arms, and gently but firmly place side body clamps to hold raised arms and head in place.
- Set upper border of lead shield with R and L markers 1-2″ (2.5-5 cm) above level of iliac crest.

Central Ray: CR ⊥, to midlung fields, mammillary (nipple) line
SID: Minimum of 72″ (183 cm)
Collimation: Collimate closely on four sides to outer chest margins.
Respiration: Full inspiration; if crying, expose at full inhalation

kV Range:	Analog: 75-80 kV			Digital Systems: 80-90 kV		
	cm	kV	mA	Time	mAs	SID	Exposure Indicator
S							
M							
L							

Bontrager Textbook, 8th ed, p. 632.

Lateral Pediatric Chest

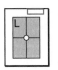

- 18 × 24 cm or 24 × 30 cm L.W. (8 × 10″ or 10 × 12″)
- TT (tabletop, nongrid) or grid with systems when it can't be removed

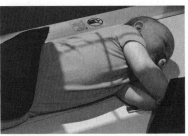

Fig. 1-21 Lateral chest (with tape and sandbags).

Position

- Lying on side, arms up with head between arms
- Support arms with tape and sandbags; ensure a true lateral.
- Flex legs; secure with tape and sandbags or with retention band across legs and hips. Lead shield over pelvic region

Central Ray: CR ⊥, to midlung fields, level of mammillary (nipple) line

SID: Minimum of 50-60″ (128-153 cm); x-ray tube raised as high as possible

Collimation: Closely collimate on four sides to outer chest margins.

Respiration: Full inspiration; if crying, time exposure at full inhalation

Note: If parental assistance is necessary, have parent hold arms overhead with head tilted back with one hand, and other hand holding down legs (provide with lead apron and gloves).

| kV Range: | Analog: 75-80 kV | | | | Digital Systems: 80-90 kV | |

	cm	kV	mA	Time	mAs	SID	Exposure Indicator
S							
M							
L							

Erect Lateral Pediatric Chest (with Pigg-O-Stat)

- 18×24 cm or 24×30 cm L.W. ($8 \times 10''$ or $10 \times 12''$)
- IR (nongrid) or grid with systems when it can't be removed

Position

- With patient remaining in same position as for PA chest, change IR and rotate entire seat and body clamps 90° into a left lateral position. Lead shield just above iliac crest
- Change lead marker to indicate left lateral.

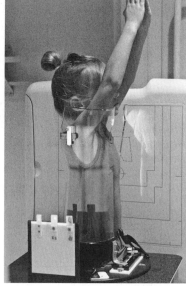

Fig. 1-22 Lateral chest (Pigg-O-Stat, for 5-year-old).

Central Ray: CR ⊥, to midlung fields, mammillary (nipple) line

SID: 72-120″ (183-307 cm)

Collimation: Closely collimate on four sides to outer chest margins.

Respiration: Full inspiration; if crying, time exposure at full inhalation

kV Range:	Analog: 75-80 kV			Digital Systems: 80-90 kV		

	cm	kV	mA	Time	mAs	SID	Exposure Indicator
S							
M							
L							

Bontrager Textbook, 8th ed., p. 634.

PA (AP) Pediatric Chest

Evaluation Criteria

Anatomy Demonstrated:
- Entire lungs from apices to costophrenic angles

Position:
- Chin elevated sufficiently
- No rotation, equal distance from lateral rib margins to spine
- Full inspiration, visualizes 9 or 10 posterior ribs above diaphragm

Exposure:
- No motion, sharp outlines of rib margins and diaphragm
- Faint outline of ribs and vertebrae through mediastinal structures

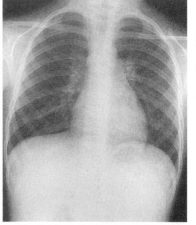

Fig. 1-23 AP (PA) pediatric chest (breathing motion is evident, blurred diaphragm, needs repeat).

Competency Check: _____
Technologist   Date

Lateral Pediatric Chest

Evaluation Criteria

Anatomy Demonstrated:
- Entire lungs from apices to costophrenic angles

Position:
- Chin and arms elevated sufficiently
- No rotation, bilateral posterior ribs superimposed

Exposure:
- No motion; sharp outline of diaphragm, rib borders, and lung markings
- Sufficient exposure to faintly visualize ribs and lung markings through heart shadow

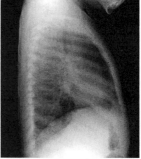

Fig. 1-24 Lateral pediatric chest (DR).

Competency Check: _____
Technologist   Date

Upper Limb (Extremity)

Pediatric Upper Limbs

(R) Routine, (S) Special

Upper Limb (Extremity)
Technical Factors

The following technical factors are important for all upper limb procedures to maximize image sharpness.

- 40-44″ (102-113 cm) SID, minimum OID
- Small focal spot
- Nongrid or TT (tabletop), detail (analog) screens
- Digital imaging requires special attention to **accurate CR and part centering** and **close collimation.**
- Short exposure time
- Immobilization (when needed)
- **Multiple exposures per imaging plate:** Multiple images can be placed on the same IP. When doing so, careful collimation and lead masking must be used to prevent pre-exposure or fogging of other images.
- **Grid use with digital systems**: Grids generally are not used with analog (film-screen) imaging for body parts measuring 10 cm or less. However, with certain digital systems, the grid may or may not be able to be removed from the receptor. In those cases, it is departmental protocol that determines if a grid is left in place or removed. **Important:** If a grid is used, the anatomy must be centered to it to avoid grid cutoff.

Radiation Protection

Collimation Close collimation is the most effective practice for preventing unnecessary radiation exposure to the patient.

Patient Shielding

Erect Patients: Patients seated at the end of the table should **always have a shield over radiosensitive organs** to prevent exposure from scatter radiation and from the divergent primary beam.

Recumbent Patients: A good practice to follow for upper limb examinations for patients on a stretcher or table is to always have shielding in place, especially the gonadal region.

Bontrager Textbook, 8th ed, pp. 136 and 137.

PA Fingers

Alternative routine: Include entire hand on PA finger projection for possible secondary trauma to other parts of hand (see PA Hand).
- 18 × 24 cm L.W. (8 × 10″)
- Nongrid
- Lead masking with multiple exposures on same IR

Position
- Patient seated at end of table, elbow flexed 90° (lead shield over lap)
- Pronate hand, separate fingers.
- Center and align long axis of affected finger(s) to portion of IR being exposed.

Central Ray: CR ⊥, centered to PIP joint

SID: 40-44″ (102-113 cm)

Collimation: On four sides to area of interest

Fig. 2-1 PA, 2nd digit.

kV Range:		Analog: 50-55 kV			Digital Systems: 55-60 kV		
	cm	kV	mA	Time	mAs	SID	Exposure Indicator
S							
M							
L							

PA Oblique Fingers

- 18 × 24 cm L.W. (8 × 10″)
- Nongrid
- Lead masking with multiple exposures on same IR

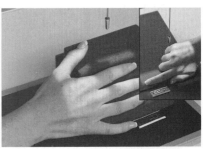

Fig. 2-2 PA oblique, 2nd digit (parallel to IR). Inset: Minimized OID.

Position
- Patient seated, hand on table, elbow flexed 90° (lead shield over lap)
- Align fingers to long axis of portion of IR being exposed.
- Rotate hand 45° medially or laterally (dependent of digit examined), resting against 45° angle support block.
- Separate fingers; ensure that affected finger(s) is (are) parallel to IR.

Central Ray: CR ⊥, centered to PIP joint

SID: 40-44″ (102-113 cm)

Collimation: On four sides to area of affected finger(s) and distal aspect of metacarpal

kV Range:	Analog: 50-55 kV			Digital Systems: 55-60 kV		

	cm	kV	mA	Time	mAs	SID	Exposure Indicator
S							
M							
L							

Bontrager Textbook, 8th ed, p. 142.

PA Finger

Evaluation Criteria

Anatomy Demonstrated:
- Distal phalanx to distal metacarpal and associated joints

Position:
- Long axis of digit parallel to IR with joints open
- No rotation of digit with symmetric appearance of shafts

Exposure:
- Optimal density and contrast (brightness and contrast for digital images)
- Soft tissue and bony trabeculation clearly demonstrated; no motion

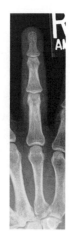

Fig. 2-3 PA finger.

Competency Check: _____
Technologist Date

Upper Limb (Extremity)

PA Oblique Finger

Evaluation Criteria

Anatomy Demonstrated:
- Distal phalanx to distal metacarpal and associated joints

Position:
- Interphalangeal and MCP joints open
- No superimposition of adjacent digits

Exposure:
- Optimal density and contrast (brightness and contrast for digital images)
- Soft tissue and bony trabeculation clearly demonstrated; no motion

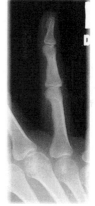

Fig. 2-4 PA oblique finger.

Competency Check: _____
Technologist Date

25

Lateral Fingers

- 18 × 24 cm
  L.W.
  (8 × 10")
- Nongrid
- Lead masking
  with multiple
  exposures on
  same IR

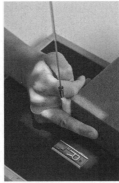

Fig. 2-5 4th digit.

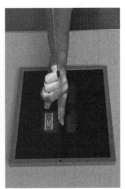

Fig. 2-6 2nd digit
(digit parallel to IR).

Position

- Patient
  seated, hand on table (lead shield over lap)
- Hand in lateral position, thumb side up for 3rd to 5th digits,
  thumb side down for 2nd digit
- Align finger to long axis of portion of IR being exposed.

Central Ray: CR ⊥, centered to PIP joint

SID: 40-44" (102-113 cm)

Collimation: On four sides to area of affected finger and distal
aspect of metacarpal

kV Range:	Analog: 50-55 kV			Digital Systems: 55-60 kV		
	cm	kV	mA	Time	mAs	SID	Exposure Indicator
S							
M							
L							

Bontrager Textbook, 8th ed, p. 143.

AP Thumb

- 18 × 24 cm L.W. (8 × 10")
- Nongrid
- Lead masking with multiple exposures on same IR

Position

- Patient standing or seated, hand rotated internally with palm out to bring the posterior surface of thumb in direct contact with IR
- Align thumb to long axis of portion of IR being exposed.

Central Ray: CR ⊥, centered to 1st MP joint

SID: 40-44" (102-113 cm)

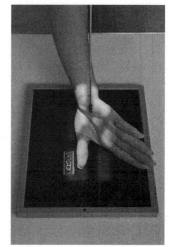

Fig. 2-7 AP thumb, CR to 1st MP joint.

Collimation: Collimate closely to area of thumb (include entire 1st metacarpal extending to carpals).

	cm	kV	mA	Time	mAs	SID	Exposure Indicator
kV Range:		Analog: 50-55 kV			Digital Systems: 55-60 kV		
S							
M							
L							

Lateral Fingers

Evaluation Criteria
Anatomy Demonstrated:
- Distal phalanx to distal metacarpal and associated joints

Position:
- True lateral: joints are open and concave appearance of anterior surfaces of shaft of phalanges

Exposure:
- Optimal density and contrast (brightness and contrast for digital images)
- Soft tissue margins and bony trabeculation clearly seen, no motion

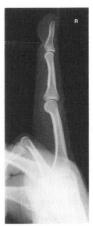

Fig. 2-8 Lateral finger.

Competency Check: _____
                   Technologist   Date

AP Thumb

Evaluation Criteria
Anatomy Demonstrated:
- Distal phalanx to proximal metacarpal and trapezium

Position:
- Long axis of thumb parallel to IR with joints open
- No rotation of thumb with symmetric appearance of shafts

Exposure:
- Optimal density and contrast (brightness and contrast for digital images)
- Soft tissue and bony trabeculation clearly demonstrated; no motion

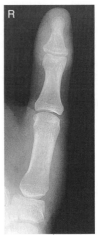

Fig. 2-9 AP thumb.

Competency Check: _____
                   Technologist   Date

PA Oblique Thumb

- 18 × 24 cm L.W. (8 × 10″)
- Nongrid
- Lead masking with multiple exposures on same IR

Position
- Patient seated, hand on table, elbow flexed (shield over lap)
- Align thumb to long axis of portion of IR being exposed.
- With hand pronated, abduct thumb slightly. This position tends to naturally rotate thumb into 45° oblique.

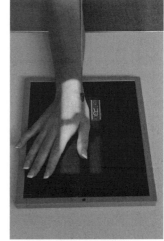

Fig. 2-10 Oblique thumb, CR to 1st MCP joint.

Central Ray: CR ⊥, centered to 1st MCP joint

SID: 40-44″ (102-113 cm)

Collimation: Collimate closely to area of thumb (include entire 1st metacarpal extending to carpals).

kV Range:	Analog: 50-55 kV			Digital Systems: 55-60 kV		
	cm	kV	mA	Time	mAs	SID	Exposure Indicator
S							
M							
L							

Lateral Thumb

- 18 × 24 cm L.W. (8 × 10″)
- Nongrid
- Lead masking with multiple exposures on same IR

Position

- Patient seated, hand on table, elbow flexed (shield across lap)
- Align thumb to long axis of portion of IR being exposed.
- With hand pronated and slightly arched, rotate hand medially until thumb is in true lateral position.

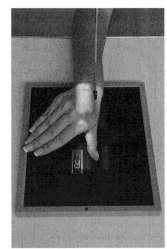

Fig. 2-11 Lateral thumb, CR to 1st MCP joint.

Central Ray: CR ⊥, centered to lst MCP joint

SID: 40-44″ (102-113 cm)

Collimation: Collimate closely to area of thumb (include entire 1st metacarpal extending to carpals).

kV Range:		Analog: 50-55 kV			Digital Systems: 55-60 kV	

	cm	kV	mA	Time	mAs	SID	Exposure Indicator
S							
M							
L							

Bontrager Textbook, 8th ed, p. 146.

PA Oblique Thumb

Evaluation Criteria
Anatomy Demonstrated:
- Distal phalanx to proximal metacarpal and trapezium

Position:
- Long axis of thumb parallel to IR with joints open

Exposure:
- Optimal density and contrast (brightness and contrast for digital images)
- Soft tissue and bony trabeculation clearly demonstrated

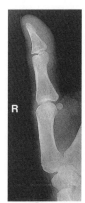

Fig. 2-12 PA oblique thumb.

Competency Check: _____
　　　　　　　　　　Technologist　　Date

Lateral Thumb

Evaluation Criteria
Anatomy Demonstrated:
- Distal phalanx to proximal metacarpal and trapezium

Position:
- True lateral position
- Interphalangeal and MCP joints open
- Anterior surfaces of first metacarpal and proximal phalanx equally concave shaped; posterior surfaces are relatively straight

Exposure:
- Optimal density and contrast (brightness and contrast for digital images)
- Soft tissue and bony trabeculation clearly demonstrated, no motion

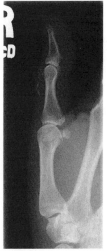

Fig. 2-13 Lateral thumb.

Competency Check: _____
　　　　　　　　　　Technologist　　Date

31

AP Axial Thumb
(Modified Roberts)

R

2

Upper Limb (Extremity)

Note: This is a special projection to better demonstrate the **first carpometacarpal joint** region.
- 18 × 24 cm L.W. (8 × 10″)
- Nongrid
- Lead masking with multiple exposures on same IR

![Fig. 2-14]

Fig. 2-14 AP axial thumb for 1st CMC joint (CR 15° proximally).

Position
- Patient seated or standing, hand rotated internally placing posterior surface of thumb directly on IR
- Align thumb to long axis of portion of IR being exposed.
- Extend fingers and hold back with other hand to prevent superimposing base of thumb and 1st CMC joint region (a key positioning requirement).

Central Ray: CR angled 15° proximally, centered to 1st CMC joint
SID: 40-44″ (102-113 cm)
Collimation: Collimate closely to entire thumb, including the trapezium carpal bone.

	cm	kV	mA	Time	mAs	SID	Exposure Indicator
kV Range:	Analog: 50-55 kV			Digital Systems: 55-60 kV			
S							
M							
L							

Bontrager Textbook, 8th ed, p. 147.

PA Hand

- 24 × 30 cm L.W. (10 × 12″)
  or
- 18 × 24 cm L.W. (8 × 10″) smaller
  hand
- Nongrid
- Lead masking with multiple
  exposures on same IR

Position
- Patient seated, hand on table,
  elbow flexed (shield
  across lap)
- Align long axis of hand and
  wrist parallel to edge of IR.
- Hand fully pronated, digits
  slightly separated

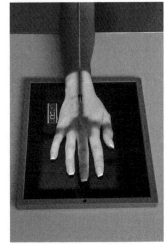

Fig. 2-15 PA hand.

Central Ray: CR ⊥, centered to 3rd MCP joint

SID: 40-44″ (102-113 cm)

Collimation: Collimate on four sides to outer margins of hand and
wrist. Include proximal and distal row of carpals.

kV Range:	Analog: 50-55 kV			Digital Systems: 55-60 kV		

	cm	kV	mA	Time	mAs	SID	Exposure Indicator
S							
M							
L							

AP Axial Thumb (Modified Roberts)

Evaluation Criteria

Anatomy Demonstrated:
- Distal phalanx to proximal metacarpal and trapezium
- Base of 1st metacarpal and trapezium well demonstrated

Position:
- Long axis of thumb parallel to IR with joints open
- No rotation

Exposure:
- Optimal density and contrast (brightness and contrast for digital images)
- Soft tissue and bony trabeculation clearly demonstrated, no motion

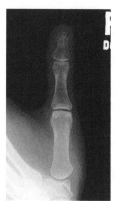

Fig. 2-16 AP axial thumb.

Competency Check: _____
Technologist   Date

PA Hand

Evaluation Criteria

Anatomy Demonstrated:
- Hand/wrist and 1″ (2.5 cm) distal forearm

Position:
- Interphalangeal and MCP joints open
- No rotation of hand with symmetric appearance of shafts of metacarpals and phalanges
- Digits slightly separated

Exposure:
- Optimal density and contrast (brightness and contrast for digital images)
- Soft tissue and bony trabeculation clearly demonstrated, no motion

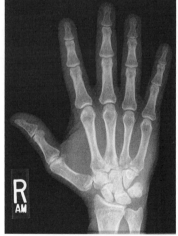

Fig. 2-17 PA hand.

Competency Check: _____
Technologist   Date

PA Oblique Hand

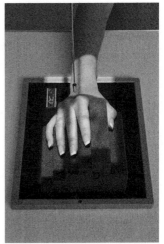

- 24 × 30 cm L.W. (10 × 12″)
  or
- 18 × 24 cm L.W. (8 × 10″) smaller
  hand
- Nongrid
- Lead masking with multiple
  exposures on same IR

Position
- Patient seated, hand on table,
  elbow flexed (shield
  across lap)
- Rotate entire hand and wrist
  laterally 45°, support with
  wedge or step block. Align
  hand and wrist to IR.

Fig. 2-18 PA oblique hand
(digits parallel to IR).

- Ensure that all digits are slightly separated and parallel to IR.

Central Ray: CR ⊥, centered to 3rd MCP joint

SID: 40-44″ (102-113 cm)

Collimation: Collimate on four sides to hand and wrist. Include
proximal and distal row of carpals.

kV Range:	Analog: 50-55 kV				Digital Systems: 55-60 kV	
	cm	kV	mA	Time	mAs	SID	Exposure Indicator
S							
M							
L							

Upper Limb (Extremity)

2

Lateral Hand (Fan and Extension Lateral)

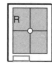

- 18 × 24 cm L.W.
  (8 × 10″)
- Nongrid
- Accessory—45°
  foam step support
- Lead masking with
  multiple exposures
  on same IR

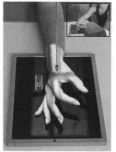

Fig. 2-19 "Fan"
lateral hand
(digits not
superimposed).

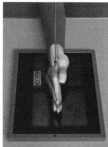

Fig. 2-20
Alternative: lateral in
extension (for
possible foreign body
and metacarpal
injury).

Position

- Patient seated,
  hand on table, elbow flexed (shield
  across lap)
- Hand in lateral position, thumb side up, digits separated and
  spread into "fan" position and supported by radiolucent step block
  or similar type support (Ensure true lateral of metacarpals.)

Central Ray: CR ⊥, centered to 2nd MCP joint

SID: 40-44″ (102-113 cm)

Collimation: Collimate on four sides to hand and wrist. Include
  proximal and distal row of carpals.

kV Range:	Analog: 60-65 kV				Digital Systems: 65-70 kV	

	cm	kV	mA	Time	mAs	SID	Exposure Indicator
S							
M							
L							

Upper Limb (Extremity)

2

R

Bontrager Textbook, 8th ed, p. 151.

PA Oblique Hand

Evaluation Criteria

Anatomy Demonstrated:
- Hand/wrist and 1″ (2.5 cm) distal forearm

Position:
- Long axis of digits/metacarpals parallel to IR with joints open
- No overlap of midshafts of 3rd to 5th metacarpals

Exposure:
- Optimal density and contrast (brightness and contrast for digital images)
- Soft tissue and bony trabeculation clearly demonstrated

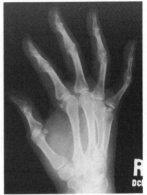

Fig. 2-21 PA oblique hand.

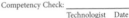
Competency Check: _____
Technologist   Date

"Fan" Lateral Hand

Evaluation Criteria

Anatomy Demonstrated:
- Hand/wrist and 1″ (2.5 cm) distal forearm
- Interphalangeal and MCP joints open

Position:
- Digits in true lateral position
- Phalanges and metacarpal surfaces symmetric
- Distal radius, ulna, and metacarpals superimposed

Exposure:
- Optimal density and contrast (brightness and contrast for digital images)
- Soft tissue and bony trabeculation clearly demonstrated

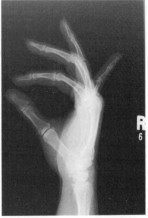

Fig. 2-22 "Fan" lateral hand.

Competency Check: _____
Technologist   Date

37

AP Oblique Bilateral Hand
(Norgaard Method and Ball-Catcher's)

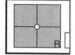

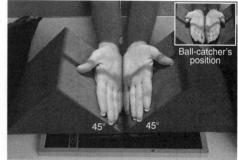

- 24 × 30 cm (10 × 12″), crosswise or 35 × 43 cm (14 × 17″) crosswise
- Nongrid
- Accessories—two 45° foam sponges for support

Fig. 2-23 AP 45° bilateral oblique. Inset: Ball-catcher's option.

Position
- Patient seated at end of table, both arms and hands extended with palms up and hands obliqued 45°, medial aspects touching
- Fingers fully extended supported by 45° support blocks

Ball-Catcher's Option:
- Fingers partially flexed, which visualizes metacarpals and MP joints well but distorts interphalangeal joints

Central Ray: CR ⊥, centered to midway between 5th MP joints
SID: 40-44″ (102-113 cm)
Collimation: Collimate to outer margins of hands and wrists. Include proximal and distal row of carpals.

kV Range:	Analog: 60-65 kV				Digital Systems: 65-70 kV	

	cm	kV	mA	Time	mAs	SID	Exposure Indicator
S							
M							
L							

Bontrager Textbook, 8th ed, p. 153.

AP Bilateral Oblique Hands (Norgaard Method)

**Evaluation
Criteria**
**Anatomy
Demonstrated:**
- Both hands from carpals to distal phalanges
- Both hands positioned in 45° oblique

Position:
- Midshafts of 2nd to 5th metacarpals not overlapped
- MCP joints open

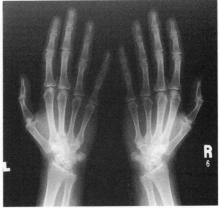

Fig. 2-24 AP bilateral oblique hand.

Competency Check: _____
Technologist   Date

Exposure:
- Optimal density and contrast (brightness and contrast for digital images)
- Soft tissue and bony trabeculation with MCP joints clearly demonstrated to distal phalanges

Upper Limb (Extremity)

PA Wrist

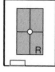

- 18 × 24 cm L.W. (8 × 10″)
- Nongrid
- Lead masking with multiple exposures on same IR

Position

- Patient seated, arm on table (shield across lap)
- Align hand and wrist parallel to edge of IR.
- Lower shoulder, rest arm on table to ensure no rotation of wrist
- Hand pronated, fingers flexed, and hand arched slightly to place wrist in direct contact with surface of IR

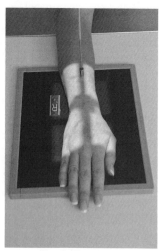

Fig. 2-25 PA wrist.

Central Ray: CR ⊥, centered to midcarpals

SID: 40-44″ (102-113 cm)

Collimation: Collimate to wrist on four sides; include distal radius and ulna and the midmetacarpal area.

kV Range:	Analog: 60-65 kV			Digital Systems: 65-70 kV		
	cm	kV	mA	Time	mAs	SID	Exposure Indicator
S							
M							
L							

Bontrager Textbook, 8th ed, p. 154.

PA Oblique Wrist

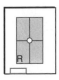

- 18 × 24 cm L.W. (8 × 10")
- Nongrid
- Lead masking with multiple exposures on same IR

Position
- Patient seated, arm on table, elbow flexed (shield across lap)
- Align hand and wrist parallel to edge of IR.
- Rotate hand and wrist laterally into 45° oblique position.

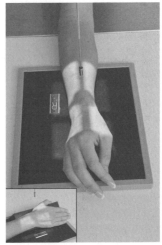

Fig. 2-26 45° PA oblique wrist.

- Flex fingers to support hand in this position, or use 45° support sponge **(inset).**

Central Ray: CR ⊥, centered to midcarpals

SID: 40-44" (102-113 cm)

Collimation: Collimate to wrist on four sides; include distal radius and ulna and the midmetacarpal area.

kV Range:	Analog: 60-65 kV			Digital Systems: 65-70 kV			
	cm	kV	mA	Time	mAs	SID	Exposure Indicator
S							
M							
L							

PA Wrist

Evaluation Criteria
Anatomy Demonstrated:
- Midmetacarpals; carpals; distal radius, ulna, and associated joints

Position:
- True PA is evidenced by symmetry of proximal metacarpals
- Separation of the distal radius and ulna

Exposure:
- Optimal density and contrast (brightness and contrast for digital images)
- Soft tissue and bony trabeculation of carpals clearly demonstrated, no motion

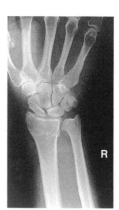

Fig. 2-27 PA wrist.

Competency Check: _____

Technologist   Date

PA Oblique Wrist

Evaluation Criteria
Anatomy Demonstrated:
- Midmetacarpals; carpals; distal radius, ulna, and associated joints

Position:
- Long axis of hand to forearm aligned to IR
- 45° oblique of wrist

Exposure:
- Optimal density and contrast (brightness and contrast for digital images)
- Soft tissue and bony trabeculation of carpals clearly demonstrated, no motion

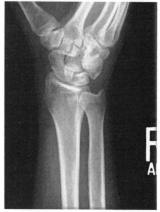

Fig. 2-28 PA oblique wrist.

Competency Check: _____

Technologist   Date

Lateral Wrist

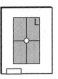

- 18 × 24 cm L.W. (8 × 10″)
- Nongrid
- Lead masking with multiple exposures on same IR

Position
- Patient seated, arm on table, elbow flexed, shoulder dropped to place humerus, forearm, and wrist on same horizontal plane
- Align hand and wrist parallel to edge of IR.
- Place hand and wrist into a true lateral position, use support to maintain this position if needed.

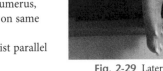

Fig. 2-29 Lateral wrist.

Central Ray: CR ⊥, centered to midcarpals

SID: 40-44″ (102-113 cm)

Collimation: Collimate to wrist on four sides; include distal radius and ulna and the midmetacarpal area.

kV Range:		Analog: 60-65 kV		Digital Systems: 65-70 kV			
	cm	kV	mA	Time	mAs	SID	Exposure Indicator
S							
M							
L							

Bontrager Textbook, 8th ed, p. 156.

Evaluation Criteria

Anatomy Demonstrated:

- Midmetacarpals; carpals; distal radius, ulna, and associated joints

Position:

- True lateral of wrist
- Ulnar head superimposed distal radius

Exposure:

- Optimal density and contrast (brightness and contrast for digital images)
- Soft tissue and bony trabeculation of carpals clearly demonstrated, no motion
- Demonstrate visible fat pads and stripes

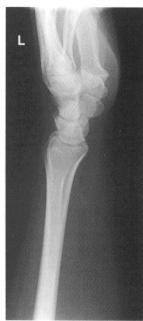

Fig. 2-30 Lateral wrist.

Competency Check: _____

Technologist   Date

PA Axial Wrist—Ulnar Deviation and Modified Stecher (Scaphoid)

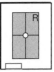

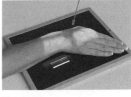

Fig. 2-31 Ulnar deviation, CR 10°-15° angle toward elbow. CR perpendicular to scaphoid.

Warning: The ulnar deviation view should be attempted only with possible wrist trauma after a routine wrist series rules out gross fractures to wrist or distal forearm. PA axial projection recommended for obscure fractures. If patient can't ulnar deviate wrist, elevate hand on 20° angle sponge.

Note: See p. 26, 8th ed textbook for joint movement terminology.

- 18 × 24 cm L.W. (8 × 10″)
- Nongrid
- Lead masking with multiple exposures on same IR

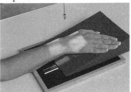

Fig. 2-32 Modified Stecher method. Elevate hand on 20° sponge, CR ⊥, to IR.

Position

- From PA wrist position, gently evert wrist toward ulnar side as far as patient can tolerate.

Central Ray: Angle CR 10°-15° proximally toward elbow, centered to scaphoid (thumb side of carpal area). If hand placed on 20° sponge, CR ⊥ to IR.

Note: A four-projection series with CR at 0°, 10°, 20°, and 30° may be required

SID: 40-44″ (102-113 cm)

Collimation: Collimate on four sides to carpal region.

	cm	kV	mA	Time	mAs	SID	Exposure Indicator
	Analog: 60-65 kV			Digital Systems: 65-70 kV			

kV Range: Analog: **60-65 kV**   Digital Systems: **65-70 kV**

	cm	kV	mA	Time	mAs	SID	Exposure Indicator
S							
M							
L							

2

Upper Limb (Extremity)

PA Axial Scaphoid (Ulnar Deviation with 15° and Modified Stecher)

Evaluation Criteria

Anatomy Demonstrated:

- Scaphoid demonstrated clearly without foreshortening or overlap
- Soft tissue and bony trabeculation of scaphoid clearly demonstrated, no motion

Position:

- Ulnar deviation evident.
- Multiple CR angles may best visualize this area.
- No rotation of wrist.

Exposure:

- Optimal density and contrast (brightness and contrast for digital images)
- Soft tissue and bony trabeculation of scaphoid clearly demonstrated, no motion

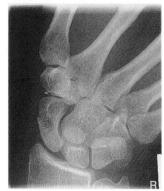

Fig. 2-33 Ulnar deviation with 15° CR angle.

Competency Check: _____
Technologist   Date

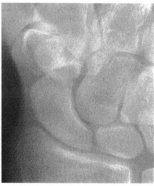

Fig. 2-34 Modified Stecher.

Competency Check: _____
Technologist   Date

PA Wrist—Radial Deviation

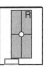

Warning: This position should be attempted for possible wrist trauma only after a routine wrist series rules out gross fractures to wrist or distal forearm.

Note: See p. 26, 8th ed textbook, for explanation on wrist joint movement terminology.

- 18 × 24 cm L.W. (8 × 10″)
- Nongrid
- Lead masking with multiple exposures on same IR

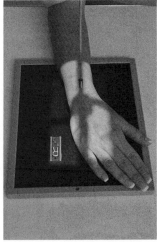

Fig. 2-35 Radial deviation, CR perpendicular. (Demonstrates ulnar side carpals.)

Position

- From PA wrist position, gently invert wrist toward radial side as far as patient can tolerate (shield across lap).

Central Ray: CR ⊥, to midcarpals

SID: 40-44″ (102-113 cm)

Collimation: Collimate closely to four sides of carpal region (≈7.5 cm or 3″ square).

kV Range:	Analog: 60-65 kV			Digital Systems: 65-70 kV		
	cm	kV	mA	Time	mAs	SID	Exposure Indicator
S							
M							
L							

PA Wrist—Radial Deviation

Evaluation Criteria

Anatomy
Demonstrated:
- Ulnar side carpals best visualized

Position:
- Radial deviation evident
- No rotation of wrist

Exposure:
- Soft tissue and bony trabeculation of ulnar aspect of carpal region clearly demonstrated, no motion

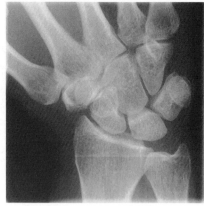

Fig. 2-36 PA wrist—radial deviation.

Competency Check: _____

Technologist　　　　　　　　Date

- Optimal density and contrast (brightness and contrast for digital images)

Wrist—Carpal Canal
(Gaynor-Hart Tangential Projection)

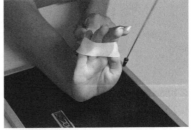

Fig. 2-37 Carpal canal (tunnel) projection (CR 25°-30° to long axis of hand).

Warning: This position is sometimes called the "tunnel view" and should be attempted for possible wrist trauma only after a routine wrist series rules out gross fractures to wrist or distal forearm.

- 18 × 24 cm L.W. (8 × 10″)
- Nongrid
- Lead masking with multiple exposures on same IR

Position
- Patient seated, hand on table (shield across lap)
- Hyperextend (dorsiflex) wrist as far as patient can tolerate with patient using other hand to hold fingers back.
- Rotate hand and wrist slightly internally—toward radius (≈5°-10°).
- Work quickly as this may be painful for patient.

Central Ray: CR 25°-30° to long axis of the palmar surface of hand, centered to ≈1″ (2-3 cm) distal to base of 3rd metacarpal

SID: 40-44″ (102-113 cm)

Collimation: Collimate to carpal region (≈7.5 cm or 3″ square).

kV Range:	Analog: 60-65 kV				Digital Systems: 65-70 kV	
	cm	kV	mA	Time	mAs	SID	Exposure Indicator
S							
M							
L							

Tangential (Gaynor-Hart) Carpal Canal

Evaluation Criteria
Anatomy Demonstrated:
- Carpals demonstrated in arched arrangement

Position:
- Pisiform and the hamular process separated
- Scaphoid/trapezium in profile

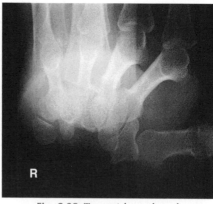

Fig. 2-38 Tangential carpal canal.

Competency Check: _____
　　　　　　　　　Technologist　　　　　　Date

Exposure:
- Optimal density and contrast (brightness and contrast for digital images)
- Soft tissues and bony trabeculation of carpal canal clearly demonstrated

AP Forearm

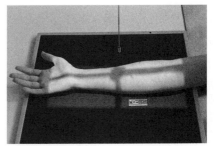

Fig. 2-39 AP forearm (to include both joints).

- 35 × 43 cm L.W. (14 × 17″) or 30 × 35 cm (11 × 14″) for smaller patients
- Nongrid
- Lead masking with multiple exposures on same IR

Position
- Patient seated at end of table with arm extended and hand supinated (shield across lap)
- Ensure that both wrist and elbow joints are included (use as large an IR as required to include both wrist and elbow joints).
- Have patient lean laterally as needed for a true AP of forearm.

Central Ray: CR ⊥, centered to midpoint of forearm

SID: 40-44″ (102-113 cm)

Collimation: Collimate on four sides, include a minimum of 2.5 cm (1″) beyond both wrist and elbow joints.

kV Range:	Analog: 60-70 kV			Digital Systems: 70-75 kV		
	cm	kV	mA	Time	mAs	SID	Exposure Indicator
S							
M							
L							

Lateral Forearm

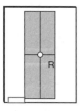

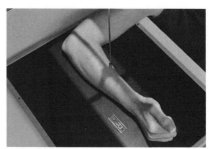

Fig. 2-40 Lateral forearm (to include both joints).

- 35 × 43 cm L.W. (14 × 17″) or 30 × 35 cm (11 × 14″) for smaller patients
- Nongrid
- Lead masking with multiple exposures on same IR

Position
- Patient seated at end of table (shield across lap)
- Elbow should be flexed 90°.
- Hand and wrist must be in a true lateral position (distal radius and ulna should be directly superimposed).
- Ensure that both wrist and elbow joints are included unless contraindicated.

Central Ray: CR ⊥, centered to midpoint of forearm

SID: 40-44″ (102-113 cm)

Collimation: Collimate on four sides, include a minimum of 2.5 cm (1″) beyond both wrist and elbow joints.

kV Range:		Analog: 60-70 kV			Digital Systems: 70-75 kV	

	cm	kV	mA	Time	mAs	SID	Exposure Indicator
S							
M							
L							

Bontrager Textbook, 8th ed., p. 163.

AP Forearm

Evaluation Criteria

Anatomy Demonstrated:
- Entire radius and ulna
- Entire elbow and proximal carpals

Position:
- Slight superimposition of proximal radius/ulna
- Humeral epicondyles in profile

Exposure:
- Optimal density and contrast (brightness and contrast for digital images)
- Soft tissues and bony trabeculation clearly demonstrated

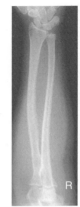

Fig. 2-41 AP forearm.

Competency Check: _____

Technologist   Date

Lateral Forearm

Evaluation Criteria

Anatomy Demonstrated:
- Entire radius and ulna demonstrated
- Entire elbow and proximal carpals demonstrated

Position:
- True lateral position
- Humeral epicondyles superimposed
- Head of ulna and distal radius are superimposed.

Exposure:
- Optimal density and contrast (brightness and contrast for digital images)
- Soft tissues and bony trabeculation of carpal canal clearly demonstrated

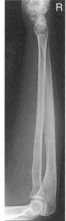

Fig. 2-42 Lateral forearm.

Competency Check: _____

Technologist   Date

53

AP Elbow

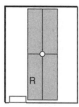

- 24 × 30 cm L.W. (10 × 12")
- Nongrid
- Lead masking with multiple exposures on same IR

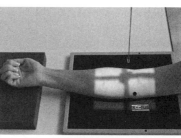

Fig. 2-43 AP, fully extended.

Position

- Elbow extended and hand supinated (shield across lap)
- Lean laterally as needed for true AP (palpate epicondyles)
- If elbow cannot be fully extended, take two AP projections as shown (Figs. 2-44 and 2-45) with CR perpendicular to distal humerus on one, and perpendicular to proximal forearm on another.

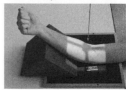

Fig. 2-44 CR, ⊥ to humerus.

Central Ray: CR ⊥, centered to mid-elbow joint

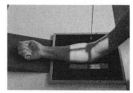

Fig. 2-45 CR ⊥ to forearm.

SID: 40-44" (102-113 cm)

Collimation: Collimate on four sides to area of interest.

	cm	kV	mA	Time	mAs	SID	Exposure Indicator
kV Range:	Analog: 60-70 kV				Digital Systems: 70-75 kV		
S							
M							
L							

Bontrager Textbook, 8th ed, pp. 164 and 165.

2

Upper Limb (Extremity)

AP Elbow—Fully Extended

Evaluation Criteria

Anatomy Demonstrated:

- Distal humerus
- Proximal radius and ulna

Position:

- Slight superimposition of proximal radius/ulna
- Humeral epicondyles in profile

Exposure:

- Optimal density and contrast (brightness and contrast for digital images)
- Soft tissues and bony trabeculation of elbow clearly demonstrated, no motion

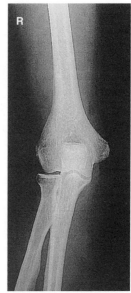

Fig. 2-46 AP elbow fully extended.

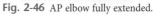

Competency Check: _____

Technologist   Date

2

Upper Limb (Extremity)

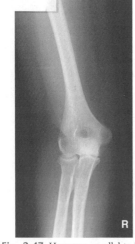

Fig. 2-47 Humerus parallel to IR.

Competency Check: _____
Technologist   Date

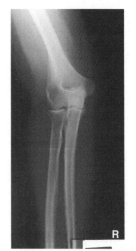

Fig. 2-48 Forearm parallel to IR.

Competency Check: _____
Technologist   Date

Evaluation Criteria

Anatomy Demonstrated:

- Distal $\frac{1}{3}$ of humerus
- Proximal $\frac{1}{3}$ of forearm

Position:

- Slight superimposition of proximal radius/ulna
- Humeral epicondyles in profile

Exposure:

- Optimal density and contrast (brightness and contrast for digital images)
- Soft tissue and bony trabeculation clearly demonstrated, no motion

Oblique Elbow (Medial and Lateral Rotation)

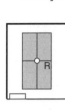

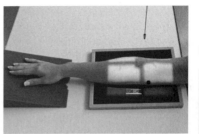

Fig. 2-49 Medial (internal) oblique (45°).

Medial (internal) oblique best visualizes coronoid process. **Lateral (external) oblique** best visualizes radial head and neck (most common oblique projection).

- 24 × 30 cm L.W. (10 × 12″)
- Nongrid

Position: Medial Oblique

- Elbow extended, hand pronated
- Palpate epicondyles to check for 45° internal rotation

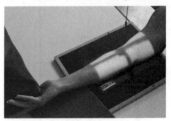

Fig. 2-50 Lateral (external) oblique (40°-45°).

Lateral Oblique: Similar position except supinate hand and rotate elbow 40°-45° externally. More difficult for patient; lean entire upper body laterally as needed.

Central Ray: CR ⊥, centered to mid-elbow joint

SID: 40-44″ (102-113 cm)

Collimation: Collimate on four sides to area of interest.

kV Range:	Analog: 60-70 kV			Digital Systems: 70-75 kV			
	cm	kV	mA	Time	mAs	SID	Exposure Indicator
S							
M							
L							

2

Upper Limb (Extremity)

Medial (Internal) Oblique Elbow

Evaluation Criteria
Anatomy Demonstrated:
- Proximal radius and ulna
- Medial epicondyle and trochlea

Position:
- Coronoid process in profile
- Radial head/neck superimposed over ulna

Exposure:
- Optimal density and contrast (brightness and contrast for digital images)
- Soft tissues and bony trabeculation clearly demonstrated

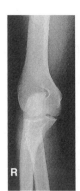

Fig. 2-51 Medial (internal) oblique elbow.

Competency Check: _____
Technologist   Date

Lateral (External) Oblique Elbow

Evaluation Criteria
Anatomy Demonstrated:
- Proximal radius and ulna
- Lateral epicondyle and capitulum

Position:
- Radial head, neck, tuberosity free of superimposition
- Humeral epicondyles and capitulum in profile

Exposure:
- Optimal density and contrast (brightness and contrast for digital images)
- Soft tissues and bony trabeculation demonstrated; no motion

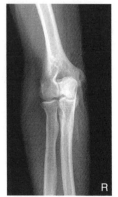

Fig. 2-52 Lateral (external) oblique elbow.

Competency Check: _____
Technologist   Date

Lateral Elbow

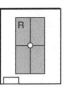

- 24 × 30 cm L.W. (10 × 12″)
- Nongrid
- Lead masking with multiple exposures on same IR

Position
- Elbow flexed 90°, shoulder dropped as needed to rest forearm and humerus flat on table and IR (shield across lap)
- Center elbow to center of IR or to portion of IR being exposed, with forearm aligned parallel to edge of cassette.
- Place hand and wrist in a true lateral position.

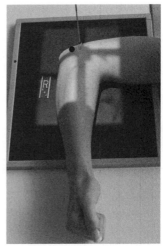

Fig. 2-53 Lateral elbow, flexed 90°.

Central Ray: CR ⊥, centered to mid-elbow joint

SID: 40-44″ (102-113 cm)

Collimation: Collimate on four sides, include a minimum of ≈5 cm (2″) of forearm and humerus.

Upper Limb (Extremity)

kV Range:	Analog: 60-70 kV			Digital Systems: 70-75 kV		
	cm	kV	mA	Time	mAs	SID	Exposure Indicator
S							
M							
L							

Lateral Elbow

Evaluation Criteria

Anatomy Demonstrated:
- Proximal radius/ulna and distal humerus
- Region of joint fat pads

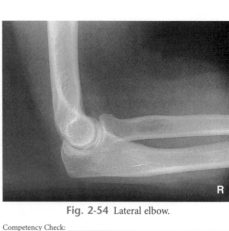

Fig. 2-54 Lateral elbow.

Competency Check: _____
Technologist   Date

Position:
- Olecranon process/ trochlear notch in profile
- Humeral epicondyles superimposed
- Elbow flexed at 90°

Exposure:
- Optimal density and contrast (brightness and contrast for digital images)
- Soft tissues and bony trabeculation clearly demonstrated

Trauma Axial Lateral Elbow
(Coyle Method)

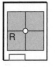

Special views to demonstrate **radial head** and **coronoid process**

- 24 × 30 cm L.W. (10 × 12″)
- Nongrid

Position and Central Ray
Radial Head and Neck:

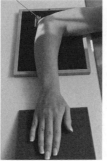

Fig. 2-55 For **radial head** and **neck**, elbow flexed **90°**.

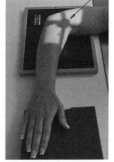

Fig. 2-56 For **coronoid process**, elbow flexed **80°**.

- Elbow flexed **90°** if possible, with hand pronated
- Angle CR 45° toward thorax, centered to radial head and neck (CR to enter at mid-elbow joint)

Coronoid Process:

- Elbow flexed **only 80°**, with hand pronated
- Angle CR 45° away from thorax, centered to coronoid process (CR to enter at mid-elbow joint)

SID: 40-44″ (102-113 cm)

Collimation: Collimate on four sides to area of interest.

| kV Range: | Analog: 65-70 kV* | | | Digital Systems: 70-75 kV | | |

	cm	kV	mA	Time	mAs	SID	Exposure Indicator
S							
M							
L							

*Increase exposure factors by 4-6 kV from lateral elbow because of angled CR.

Upper Limb (Extremity)

2

Trauma Axial Lateral Elbow
(Coyle Method)

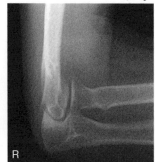

Fig. 2-57 Axial lateral elbow (for radial head, neck, and capitulum).

Competency Check: _____
Technologist   Date

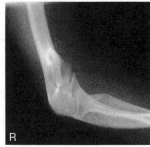

Fig. 2-58 Axial lateral elbow (for coronoid process and trochlea).

Competency Check: _____
Technologist   Date

Evaluation Criteria

Anatomy Demonstrated and Position—CR 45° Toward Shoulder:
- Radial head, neck, and capitulum; elbow flexed **90°**

Anatomy Demonstrated and Position—CR 45° Away from Shoulder:
- Coronoid process and trochlea
- Coronoid process in profile, elbow flexed **80°** (Flexion of more than 80° will obscure coronoid process)

Exposure:
- Optimal density and contrast (brightness and contrast for digital images)
- Soft tissues and bony trabeculation clearly demonstrated; no motion

Pediatric AP Upper Limb

With possible trauma, handle limb very gently with minimal movement. Take a single exposure to rule out gross fractures before additional radiographs are taken.

Fig. 2-59 AP, upper limb.

- IR size determined by patient age and size
- TT (tabletop IR) or image receptor

Position

- Supine position, arm abducted away from body, lead shield over pelvic area
- Include entire limb unless a specific joint or bone is indicated.
- Immobilize with clear flexible-type retention band and sandbags, or with tape.
- Use parental assistance only if necessary, provide lead gloves and apron.

Central Ray: CR ⊥, centered to midlimb
SID: 40-44" (102-113 cm)
Collimation: On four sides to area of interest

Upper Limb (Extremity)

kV Range:		Analog and Digital Systems: **50-65 kV**				
	cm	kV	mA	Time	mAs	SID	Exposure Indicator
S							
M							
L							

Pediatric Lateral Upper Limb

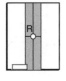

- IR size determined by patient age and size
- TT (detail screens) or DR image receptor

Position

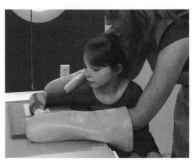

Fig. 2-60 Lateral, upper limb.

- Supine position with arm abducted away from body, lead shield over pelvic area
- Include entire limb unless a specific joint or bone is indicated.
- Immobilize with clear flexible-type retention band and sandbags or with tape.
- Flex elbow and rotate entire arm into a lateral position.
- Use parental assistance only if necessary, provide lead gloves and apron.

Central Ray: CR ⊥, centered to midlimb

SID: 40-44″ (102-113 cm)

Collimation: On four sides to area of interest

kV Range:				Analog and Digital Systems: 50-60 kV		
	cm	kV	mA	Time	mAs	SID	Exposure Indicator
S							
M							
L							

Bontrager Textbook, 8th ed, p. 635.

Chapter 3

Humerus and Shoulder Girdle

Important for humerus and shoulder projections: Do not attempt to rotate upper limb if fracture or dislocation is suspected without special orders by a physician.

(R) Routine, (S) Special

Humerus and Shoulder Girdle

AP Humerus

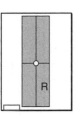

- 35 × 43 cm L.W. (14 × 17″) or for small patient 30 × 35 cm L.W. (11 × 14″)
- Grid >10 cm, IR only <10 cm
- Lead masking

Position

- Erect or supine with humerus aligned to long axis of IR (unless diagonal placement is needed to **include both elbow and shoulder joints**). Place shield over gonads.
- Abduct arm slightly, supinate hand for true AP (epicondyles parallel to IR)

Central Ray: CR ⊥, to midhumerus

SID: 40-44″ (102-113 cm)

Collimation: Collimate on sides to soft tissue borders of humerus and shoulder.

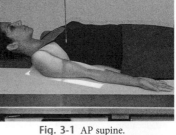

Fig. 3-1 AP supine.

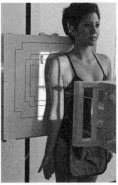

Fig. 3-2 AP erect.

	cm	kV	mA	Time	mAs	SID	Exposure Indicator
kV Range:	Analog: 70 ± 6 kV				Digital Systems: 75-80 kV		
S							
M							
L							

Rotational Lateral Humerus

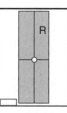

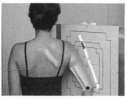

Fig. 3-3 Erect lateral (PA).

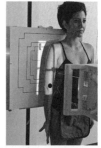

Fig. 3-4 Erect lateral (AP).

Warning: Do not attempt to rotate arm if fracture or dislocation is suspected (see following page).
- 35 × 43 cm L.W. (14 × 17″) or 30 × 35 cm L.W.
- Grid >10 cm, IR only <10 cm

Position (May Be Taken Erect AP or PA, or Supine)
- **Erect (PA):** Elbow flexed 90°, patient rotated 15°-20° from PA or as needed to bring humerus and shoulder in contact with IR holder (epicondyles ⊥ to IR for true lateral)

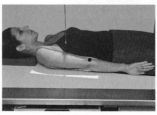

Fig. 3-5 Supine lateral.

- **Erect or supine AP:** Elbow slightly flexed, arm and wrist rotated for lateral position (palm back), epicondyles ⊥ to IR
- IR centered to **include both elbow and shoulder joints**

Central Ray: CR ⊥, to midhumerus

SID: 40-44″ (102-113 cm)

Collimation: Collimate on sides to soft tissue borders of humerus and shoulder

				Analog: 70 ± 6 kV		Digital Systems: 75-80 kV	

kV Range: Analog: 70 ± 6 kV   Digital Systems: 75-80 kV

	cm	kV	mA	Time	mAs	SID	Exposure Indicator
S							
M							
L							

Bontrager Textbook, 8th ed., p. 184.

Trauma Lateral Humerus
(Midhumerus and Distal Humerus)

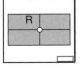

For proximal humerus, see transthoracic lateral or scapular Y.

- 30 × 35 cm L.W. (11 × 14″) or 24 × 30 cm L.W. (10 × 12″)
- Nongrid

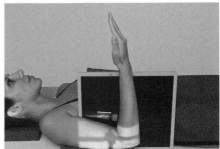

Fig. 3-6 Lateral cross-table, midhumerus and distal humerus.

Position

- Gently lift arm and place support block under arm, rotate hand into lateral position if possible for true lateral elbow projection
- Place IR vertically between arm and thorax with top of IR at axilla (place shield between IR and patient)

Central Ray: CR horizontal and ⊥ to IR, centered to distal $\frac{1}{3}$ of humerus

SID: 40-44″ (102-113 cm)

Collimation: Collimate on four sides, include distal and midhumerus, elbow joint, and proximal forearm

	kV Range:	Analog: 64 ± 6 kV		Digital Systems: 70-80 kV		
	cm	kV	mA	Time	mAs	SID	Exposure Indicator
S							
M							
L							

AP and Lateral Humerus

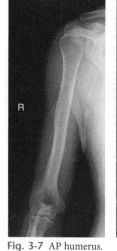

Fig. 3-7 AP humerus.

Competency Check: _____
              Technologist   Date

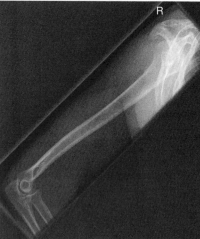

Fig. 3-8 Lateral erect humerus.

Competency Check: _____
              Technologist   Date

Evaluation Criteria

Anatomy Demonstrated:

- AP and lateral view of the entire humerus, including elbow and glenohumeral joints

Position: AP

- No rotation, medial and lateral epicondyles seen in profile, greater tubercle in profile laterally
- Humeral head and glenoid cavity demonstrated

Lateral (PA)

- True lateral, epicondyles are directly superimposed

Exposure:

- Optimal density (brightness) and contrast
- Sharp bony trabeculation clearly demonstrated, no motion

Trauma Transthoracic Lateral Humerus
(Midhumerus and Proximal Humerus)

- 35 × 43 cm L.W.
  (14 × 17″)
- Grid

Position
- Patient recumbent or erect
- Affected limb closest to IR
- Raise opposite arm over head

Fig. 3-9 Transthoracic lateral.

Central Ray: Center to mid-shaft of affected humerus

SID: 40-44″ (102-113 cm)

Collimation: To soft tissue margins—entire humerus

Respiration: Breathing technique is preferred.

If breathing lateral technique performed: Minimum of 2 seconds exposure time (between 2 and 4 seconds is desirable)

kV Range:	Analog: 75-75 kV		Digital Systems: 75-80 kV			
	cm	kV	mA	Time	mAs	SID	Exposure Indicator
S							
M							
L							

Transthoracic Lateral Proximal Humerus

Evaluation Criteria

Anatomy Demonstrated:

- Lateral view of the proximal half of humerus

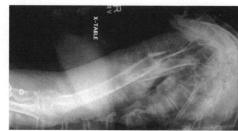

Fig. 3-10 Transthoracic lateral.

Position:

- Proximal half of shaft of humerus should be clearly visualized
- Humeral head and glenoid cavity demonstrated

Competency Check: _____

                      Technologist   Date

Exposure:

- Optimal density (brightness) and contrast
- Overlying ribs and lung markings blurred (with breathing technique)

Humerus and Shoulder Girdle

AP Shoulder
(External and Internal Rotation)

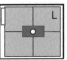

Warning: Do not attempt if fracture or dislocation is suspected.

- 24 × 30 cm (10 × 12″) C.W. (or lengthwise to show more of humerus)
- Grid

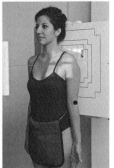

Fig. 3-11 External (AP humerus).

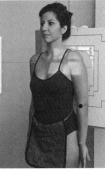

Fig. 3-12 Internal (lateral humerus).

Humerus and Shoulder Girdle

Position
- Erect (seated or standing) or supine, arm slightly abducted
- Rotate thorax as needed to place posterior shoulder against IR
- Center of IR to scapulohumeral joint and CR

External Rotation: Rotate arm externally until hand is supinated and epicondyles are parallel to IR.

Internal Rotation: Rotate arm internally until hand is pronated and epicondyles are perpendicular to IR.

Central Ray: CR ⊥, directed to 1″ (2.5 cm) inferior to coracoid process

SID: 40-44″ (102-113 cm)

Collimation: Collimate closely on four sides.

Respiration: Suspend during exposure.

| kV Range: | Analog: 70-75 kV | | | | Digital Systems: 75-80 kV | |

	cm	kV	mA	Time	mAs	SID	Exposure Indicator
S							
M							
L							

Bontrager Textbook, 8th ed, pp. 187 and 188.

AP Shoulder—External and Internal Rotation

Evaluation Criteria
Anatomy
Demonstrated:
- Proximal humerus and lateral $^2/_3$ of the clavicle (entire clavicle for crosswise IR) and upper scapula

Position: External Rotation
- Greater tubercle visualized in full profile laterally
- Lesser tubercle superimposed over humeral head

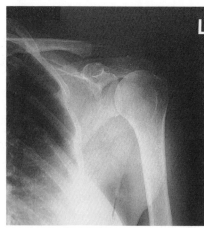

Fig. 3-13 AP shoulder external rotation.

Competency Check: _____
Technologist   Date

Internal Rotation (Lateral)
- Lesser tubercle visualized in full profile medially
- Greater tubercle superimposed over humeral head

Exposure:
- Optimal density (brightness) and contrast
- Soft tissue and sharp bony trabeculation clearly demonstrated; no motion

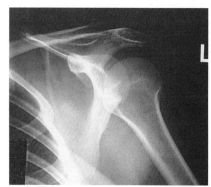

Fig. 3-14 AP shoulder internal rotation.

Competency Check: _____
Technologist   Date

Humerus and Shoulder Girdle

Inferosuperior Axial
(Lawrence Method)

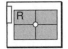

Warning: Do not attempt if fracture or dislocation is suspected.

- 18 × 24 cm C.W. (8 × 10″)
- Grid; grid lines horizontal and CR to center line of grid
- Often performed nongrid for smaller shoulder

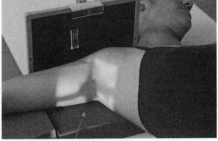

Fig. 3-15 Inferosuperior axial (Lawrence method).

Position

- Patient supine, to front edge of table or stretcher, with support under shoulder to center anatomy to IR, head turned away from IR
- Arm abducted 90° from body if possible
- Rotate arm externally, with hand supinated

Central Ray: CR horizontal, directed 25°-30° medially to axilla, less angle if arm is not abducted 90° (place tube next to table or stretcher at same level as axilla)

SID: 40-44″ (102-113 cm)

Collimation: Collimate closely on four sides

Respiration: Suspend during exposure

| kV Range: | Analog: 70-75 kV | | | Digital Systems: 75-80 kV | | |

	cm	kV	mA	Time	mAs	SID	Exposure Indicator
S							
M							
L							

Humerus and Shoulder Girdle

3

Inferosuperior Axial
(Lawrence Method)

Evaluation Criteria

Anatomy Demonstrated:

- Lateral view of proximal humerus in relationship to the glenoid fossa

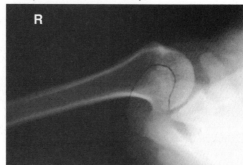

Fig. 3-16 Inferosuperior axial (Lawrence method).

Competency Check: _____
Technologist   Date

Position:

- Spine of scapula is seen in profile inferior to the scapulohumeral joint.
- Affected arm abducted about 90°

Exposure:

- Optimal density (brightness) and contrast
- Soft tissue and sharp bony trabeculation clearly demonstrated; no motion

Humerus and Shoulder Girdle

PA Transaxillary Projection
(Hobbs Modification)

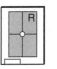

- 18 × 24 cm L.W. (8 × 10″)
- Grid

Position
- Patient recumbent or erect PA
- Affected arm raised superiorly
- Head is turned away

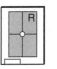

Fig. 3-17 PA transaxillary (Hobbs modification).

Central Ray: Perpendicular to the IR, centered to the glenohumeral joint

SID: 40-44″ (102-113 cm)

Collimation: Collimate closely on four sides.

Respiration: Suspend during exposure.

3

Humerus and Shoulder Girdle

kV Range:		Analog: 70-75 kV		Digital Systems: 75-80 kV		
	cm	kV	mA	Time	mAs	SID	Exposure Indicator
S							
M							
L							

PA Transaxillary Projection
(Hobbs Modification)

Evaluation Criteria
Anatomy Demonstrated:
- Lateral view of proximal humerus in relationship to glenohumeral joint

Position:
- Coracoid process of scapula is seen on end
- Affected arm elevated completely

Exposure:
- Optimal density (brightness) and contrast
- Soft tissue and sharp bony trabeculation clearly demonstrated; no motion

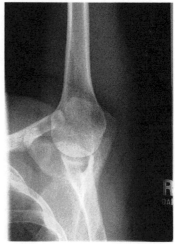

Fig. 3-18 PA transaxillary (Hobbs modification).

Competency Check: _____

Technologist   Date

Inferosuperior Axial
(Clements Modification)

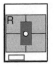

- 18 × 24 cm L.W. (8 × 10")
- Nongrid (can use grid if CR is perpendicular to it)

Position
- Lateral recumbent position
- Affected arm up
- Abduct arm 90° from body if possible.

Central Ray: Direct horizontal CR perpendicular to the IR.

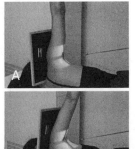

Fig. 3-19 Inferosuperior axial (Clements modification).

(Angle the tube 5°-15° toward the axilla if the patient cannot abduct the arm 90°)

SID: 40-44" (102-113 cm)

Collimation: Collimate closely on four sides.

Respiration: Suspend during exposure.

Humerus and Shoulder Girdle

3

kV Range: Analog: 70-75 kV   Digital Systems: 75-80 kV

	cm	kV	mA	Time	mAs	SID	Exposure Indicator
S							
M							
L							

Inferosuperior Axial
(Clements Modification)

Evaluation Criteria

Anatomy Demonstrated:

- Lateral view of proximal humerus in relationship to the scapulohumeral joint

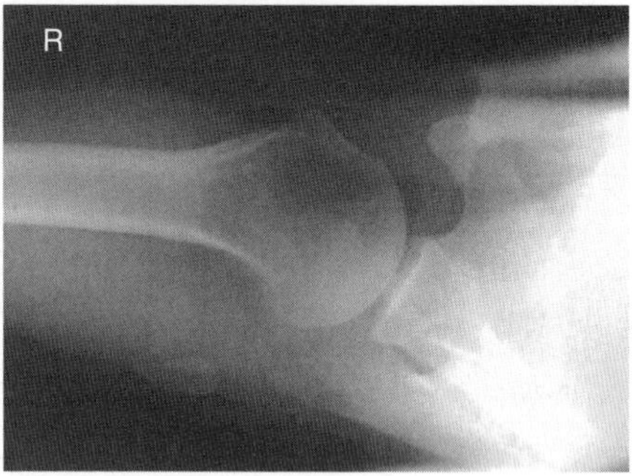

Fig. 3-20 Inferosuperior axial (Clements modification).

Competency Check: _____

Technologist   Date

Position:

- Arm is abducted 90° from the body.

Exposure:

- Optimal density (brightness) and contrast
- Soft tissue and sharp bony trabeculation clearly demonstrated; no motion

Posterior Oblique
(Grashey Method)

A special projection for visualizing glenoid cavity in profile with open joint space
- 18 × 24 cm C.W. (8 × 10")
- Grid

Fig. 3-21 Glenoid cavity (35°-45° post. oblique).

Position

- Erect or supine (erect preferred)
- Oblique 35°-45° toward side of interest (body of scapula should be parallel with IR), hand and arm in neutral rotation
- Center scapulohumeral joint and IR to CR (2" [5 cm] inferior and medial from the superolateral border of shoulder)

Central Ray: CR ⊥, to midscapulohumeral joint

SID: 40-44" (102-113 cm)

Collimation: Collimate so upper and lateral borders of the field are to the soft tissue margins.

Respiration: Suspend during exposure.

kV Range:	Analog: 70-75 kV				Digital Systems: 75-80 kV	
	cm	kV	mA	Time	mAs	SID	Exposure Indicator
S							
M							
L							

Posterior Oblique
(Grashey Method)

Evaluation Criteria
Anatomy Demonstrated:
- View of head of humerus in relationship to glenoid cavity

Position:
- Open scapulohumeral joint space
- Anterior and posterior rims of glenoid cavity are superimposed

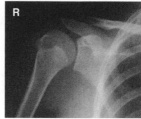

Fig. 3-22 Posterior oblique.

Competency Check: _____
Technologist   Date

Exposure:
- Optimal density (brightness) and contrast
- Soft tissue and sharp bony trabeculation clearly demonstrated; no motion

Humerus and Shoulder Girdle

Tangential Projection—Intertubercular (Bicipital) Groove

(Fisk Modification)

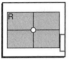

- 18 × 24 cm C.W. (8 × 10″)
- Nongrid

Position

- Supine or erect. Palpate anterior humeral head to locate groove.

Supine: Abduct arm slightly, supinate hand.

- Center IR and groove to CR.
- CR 10°-15° down from horizontal position of x-ray tube, centered to groove, IR vertical against top of shoulder, perpendicular to CR

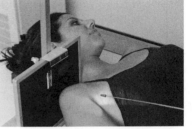

Fig. 3-23 Supine inferosuperior projection (CR 15°-20° from horizontal).

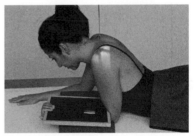

Fig. 3-24 Erect superoinferior (humerus 15°-20° from vertical, CR, ⊥ to IR).

Alternative Erect: Patient leans forward 15°-20°, CR vertical, ⊥ to IR

SID: 40-44″ (102-113 cm)

Collimation: Collimate closely on four sides to area of anterior humeral head.

Respiration: Suspend during exposure.

kV Range:		Analog: 60-65 kV		Digital Systems: 65-75 kV			
	cm	kV	mA	Time	mAs	SID	Exposure Indicator
S							
M							
L							

Humerus and Shoulder Girdle

3

Tangential Projection Intertubercular (Bicipital) Groove

(Fisk Modification)

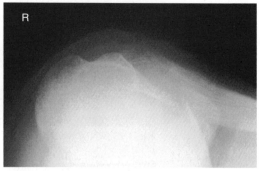

Fig. 3-25 Tangential projection (intertubercular groove).

Competency Check: _____

Technologist   Date

Evaluation Criteria

Anatomy Demonstrated:
- Humeral tubercles and intertubercular groove seen in profile

Position:
- Intertubercular groove and tubercles in profile
- No superimposition of acromion process

Exposure:
- Optimal density (brightness) and contrast
- Soft tissue and sharp bony trabeculation clearly demonstrated; no motion

Scapular Y Lateral—Anterior Oblique Position and Neer Method

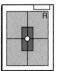

- 24 × 30 cm L.W. (10 × 12″)
- Grid

Position
- Erect or recumbent (erect preferred)
- Rotate patient into a 45°-60° anterior oblique as for a lateral scapula (body of scapula perpendicular to IR).
- Unaffected arm up in front of patient, affected arm down (**don't move with possible fracture or dislocation**)
- Center scapulohumeral joint and CR.

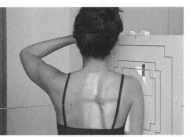

Fig. 3-26 Scapular Y lateral position—CR ⊥.

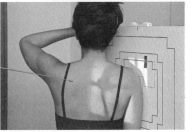

Fig. 3-27 Neer method—CR 10°-15° caudad.

Central Ray: CR ⊥ to scapulohumeral joint

Neer Method: Angle CR 10°-15° caudad to better demonstrate the acromiohumeral space (supraspinatus outlet), CR to superior margin of humeral head

SID: 40-44″ (102-113 cm)

Collimation: Collimate on four sides to area of interest.

Respiration: Suspend during exposure.

kV Range:	Analog: 70-75 kV			Digital Systems: 75-80 kV		
	cm	kV	mA	Time	mAs	SID	Exposure Indicator
S							
M							
L							

Humerus and Shoulder Girdle

3

Scapular Y Lateral—Anterior Oblique Position and Neer Method

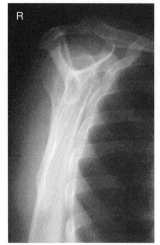

Fig. 3-28 Scapular Y projection.

Competency Check: _____
                 Technologist   Date

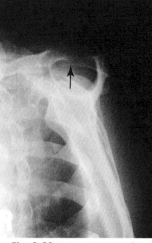

Fig. 3-29 Supraspinatus outlet projection (Neer method).

Competency Check: _____
                 Technologist   Date

Evaluation Criteria

Anatomy Demonstrated:

- **Scapular Y:** True lateral view of the scapula, proximal humerus
- **Neer method:** Supraspinatus outlet region is open

Position:

- **Scapular Y:** Thin body of the scapula seen on end without rib superimposition. Upper limb is not elevated or moved with possible fracture or dislocation.
- **Neer method:** Thin body of the scapula seen on end; humeral head below supraspinatus outlet *(arrow)*

Exposure:

- Optimal density (brightness) and contrast
- Soft tissue and sharp bony trabeculation clearly demonstrated; no motion

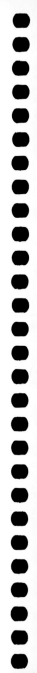

AP Shoulder Trauma Projection
(Neutral Rotation)

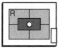

- 24 × 30 cm C.W. (10 × 12″) (or lengthwise to show more of humerus if injury includes proximal half of humerus)
- Grid

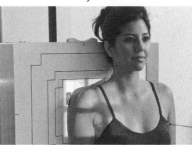

Fig. 3-30 AP—neutral rotation.

Note: Evaluation of AP shoulder-neutral position is similar to external/internal rotation, but neither the greater nor lesser tubercle is in profile (if limb can be moved).

Position

- Erect (seated or standing) or supine, arm slightly abducted
- Rotate thorax slightly as needed to place posterior shoulder against IR
- Arm in neutral position (generally this is with palm inward—no acute trauma present)

Central Ray: CR ⊥, to ≈2-3 cm (1″) inferior to coracoid process

SID: 40-44″ (102-113 cm)

Collimation: Collimate on four sides to area of interest.

Respiration: Suspend during exposure.

| kV Range: | Analog: 70-75 kV | | | Digital Systems: 75-85 kV | | |

	cm	kV	mA	Time	mAs	SID	Exposure Indicator
S							
M							
L							

Lateral Shoulder Trauma Projection
Transthoracic Lateral (Lawrence Method)

- 24 × 30 cm L.W. (10 × 12″)
- Grid
- Breathing technique is preferred if patient can cooperate

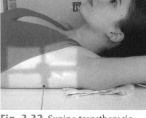

Fig. 3-31 Erect transthoracic lateral.

Position
- Erect or supine, affected arm against IR, arm at side in neutral position
- Raise unaffected arm above head.
- Elevate unaffected shoulder, **or** angle CR 10°-15° cephalad to prevent superimposition of unaffected shoulder.
- True lateral, or slight anterior rotation of unaffected shoulder
- Center grid IR to CR.

Fig. 3-32 Supine transthoracic lateral.

Central Ray: CR ⊥, through thorax to surgical neck

SID: 40-44″ (102-113 cm)

Collimation: Collimate on four sides to area of interest.

Respiration: 3-4 sec with breathing technique or suspended respiration

kV Range:	Analog: 70-75 kV				Digital Systems: 75-80 kV	

	cm	kV	mA	Time	mAs	SID	Exposure Indicator
S							
M							
L							

Bontrager Textbook, 8th ed, p. 195.

Transthoracic Lateral Shoulder Projection
(Lawrence Method)

Evaluation Criteria

Anatomy Demonstrated:

- Lateral view of proximal humerus and glenohumeral joint

Position:

- Shaft of the proximal humerus should be clearly visualized
- Humeral head and the glenoid cavity visualized

Exposure:

- Optimal density (brightness) and contrast
- Soft tissue and sharp bony trabeculation clearly demonstrated; no motion

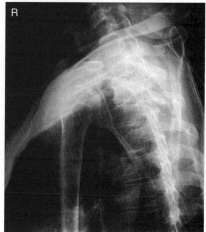

Fig. 3-33 Transthoracic lateral.

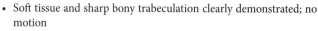

Competency Check: _____

          Technologist   Date

3

Humerus and Shoulder Girdle

AP Apical Oblique Axial Shoulder
(Garth Method)

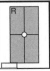

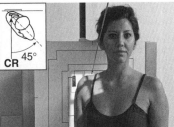

Fig. 3-34 Erect apical oblique (45° posterior obli., CR 45° caudad).

A good projection for acute shoulder trauma, demonstrating shoulder dislocations, glenoid fractures, and Hill-Sachs lesions
- 24 × 30 cm L.W. (10 × 12″)
- Grid

Humerus and Shoulder Girdle

Position
- Erect preferred (recumbent if necessary)
- Rotate thorax 45° with affected shoulder against IR
- Flex affected elbow and place hand on opposite shoulder
- Center IR to exiting CR

Central Ray: CR 45° caudad, to medial aspect of scapulohumeral joint

SID: 40-44″ (102-113 cm)

Collimation: Collimate on four sides to area of interest.

Respiration: Suspend during exposure.

kV Range:	Analog: 75-75 kV			Digital Systems: 75-80 kV		

	cm	kV	mA	Time	mAs	SID	Exposure Indicator
S							
M							
L							

Bontrager Textbook, 8th ed, p. 198.

AP Apical Oblique Axial Projection
(Garth Method)

Evaluation Criteria
Anatomy Demonstrated:
- Humeral head, glenoid cavity, and neck and head of scapula free of superimposition

Position:
- Acromion and AC joint projected superior to humeral head

Exposure:
- Optimal density (brightness) and contrast
- Soft tissue and sharp bony trabeculation clearly demonstrated; no motion

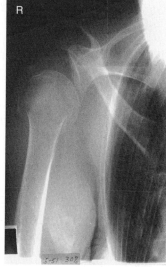

Fig. 3-35 AP apical oblique.

Competency Check: _____
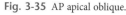
                           Technologist   Date

Humerus and Shoulder Girdle

AP and AP Axial Clavicle

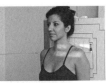

Fig. 3-36 AP, 0°.

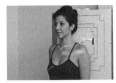

Fig. 3-37 AP axial, 20° cephalad.

- 24 × 30 cm C.W. (10 × 12″)
- Grid

Position

- Erect or recumbent
- Center clavicle and IR to CR (midway between jugular notch medially and AC joint laterally)

Central Ray: CR to midclavicle

AP: CR ⊥, to midclavicle

AP Axial: 15°-30° cephalad* (thin shoulders require 5°-10° more angle than thick shoulders)

Note: Departmental routines may include AP 0°, or axial AP, or both.

SID: 40-44″ (102-113 cm)

Collimation: Collimate to area of clavicle. (Ensure that both AC and sternoclavicular joints are included.)

Respiration: Expose upon full inspiration.

*AP lordotic position can be performed rather than angling CR for AP axial.

kV Range:	Analog: **75-75 kV** (+4 kV for axial)	Digital Systems: **75-80 kV**

	cm	kV	mA	Time	mAs	SID	Exposure Indicator
S							
M							
L							

AP and AP Axial Clavicle Projection

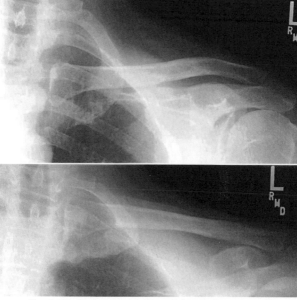

Fig. 3-38 AP clavicle and AP axial clavicle (lower image).

Competency Check: _____

Technologist   Date

Evaluation Criteria

Anatomy Demonstrated:

- **AP 0°:** Entire clavicle
- **AP axial:** The clavicle above the scapula and ribs

Position:

- **AP 0°:** Entire clavicle from AC to SC joint
- **AP axial:** Only medial portion of clavicle will be superimposed by 1st and 2nd ribs.

Exposure:

- Optimal density (brightness) and contrast
- Soft tissue and sharp bony trabeculation clearly demonstrated; no motion

93

AP Scapula

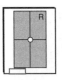

- 24 × 30 cm L.W.
  (10 × 12″)
- Grid

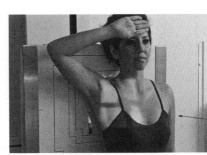

Fig. 3-39 AP scapula.

Position

- Erect or supine
  (erect preferred with
  pain in scapula area)
- Gently abduct arm 90° if possible, supinate hand (abduction
  results in less superimposition of scapula by ribs).
- Center IR and entire scapula to CR.

Central Ray: CR ⊥, to midscapula (≈5 cm or 2″ inferior to coracoid
  process and ≈2-3 cm [1″] medial to lateral border)

SID: 40-44″ (102-113 cm)

Collimation: Collimate on four sides of scapula borders.

Respiration: Breathing technique can be employed or suspend
  during exposure.

kV Range:		Analog: 75-75 kV		Digital Systems: 75-80 kV		

	cm	kV	mA	Time	mAs	SID	Exposure Indicator
S							
M							
L							

Bontrager Textbook, 8th ed, p. 202.

Lateral Scapula

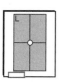

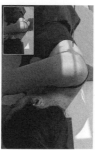

- 24 × 30 cm
  L.W.
  (10 × 12″)

Fig. 3-40 Lateral (palpate scapular borders).

Position

- Erect or recumbent (erect preferred)
- Palpate borders of scapula and rotate thorax until body of scapula is perpendicular to IR (will vary from 45°-60° rotation).
- If area of interest is body of scapula, with arm up have patient reach across and grasp opposite shoulder.

Central Ray: CR ⊥, to mid-medial (vertebral) border

SID: 40-44″ (102-113 cm)

Collimation: To scapular region

Respiration: Suspend during exposure.

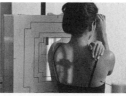

Fig. 3-41 For body of scapula.

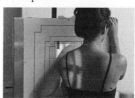

Fig. 3-42 Superior scapula (acromion or coracoid process), place arm down, flex elbow, palm out.

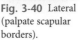

Humerus and Shoulder Girdle

3

	kV Range:	Analog: 75-80 kV		Digital Systems: 75-80 kV			
	cm	kV	mA	Time	mAs	SID	Exposure Indicator
S							
M							
L							

AP and Lateral Scapula Projections

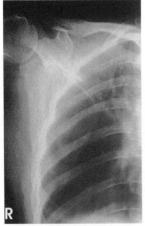

Fig. 3-43 AP scapula.

Competency Check: _____
Technologist   Date

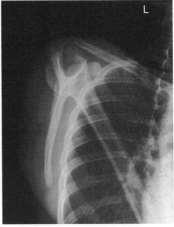

Fig. 3-44 Lateral scapula.

Competency Check: _____
Technologist   Date

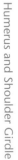
Evaluation Criteria

Anatomy Demonstrated:

- **AP:** Entire scapula
- **Lateral:** Entire scapula in a lateral position

Position:

- **AP:** Lateral border of scapula free of superimposition
- **Lateral:** Humerus not superimposing over region of interest; ribs free of superimposition by body of scapula

Exposure:

- Optimal density (brightness) and contrast
- Soft tissue and sharp bony trabeculation clearly demonstrated; no motion

Acromioclavicular (AC) Joints

(AP—Bilateral with and without Weights)

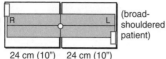

18 cm (8") | R   L | (broad-shouldered patient)

24 cm (10")   24 cm (10")

Warning: Rule out fracture first before taking "with weight" projection.

- 35 × 43 cm C.W. (14 × 17") or (2) 18 × 24 cm (8 × 10") for broad shoulders
- Grid or nongrid (depending on size of shoulder)
- Use markers "with weights" and "without weights"

Position

- Erect, standing if possible, or may be seated on chair
- Arms at sides, one exposure for bilateral without weights, and a second exposure with 8-10 lb (5-8 lb for smaller patient) weights tied to wrists, shoulders and arms relaxed, center IR to CR

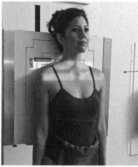

Fig. 3-45 Bilateral with weights.

Central Ray: CR ⊥, to jugular notch

SID: 72-120" (183-307 cm)

Collimation: Long, narrow horizontal exposure field

Respiration: Suspend during exposure.

kV Range:		Analog: **65-70 kV**			Digital Systems: **70-80 kV**		

	cm	kV	mA	Time	mAs	SID	Exposure Indicator
S							
M							
L							

AP AC Joint Projections—Bilateral with and without Weights

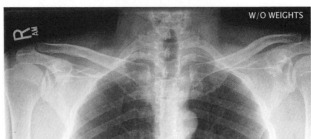

Fig. 3-46 AC joints without weights.

Competency Check: _____

Technologist   Date

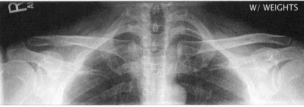

Fig. 3-47 AC joints with weights.

Competency Check: _____

Technologist   Date

Evaluation Criteria

Anatomy Demonstrated:

- Both R and L AC joints and SC joints included

Position:

- No rotation, symmetric SC joints

Exposure:

- Optimal density (brightness) and contrast; no motion
- Soft tissue and sharp bony trabeculation clearly demonstrated

Chapter 4

Lower Limb (Extremity)

4

Lower Limb (Extremity)

(R) Routine, (S) Special

Lower Limb (Extremity)

Technical Considerations

The principal exposure factors for radiography of the lower limbs include the following:

- Low-to-medium kV (50-70); digital radiography permits for higher kV
- Short exposure time
- Small focal spot
- Adequate mAs for sufficient density (brightness)
- Detail (analog) intensifying screens commonly used
- Grids: for anatomy measuring greater than 10 cm in thickness

Digital Imaging Considerations

- **Four-sided collimation:** Collimate to the area of interest with a minimum of two collimation parallel borders clearly demonstrated on the image. Four-sided collimation is always preferred if study allows it.
- **Accurate centering:** It is important that the body part and the central ray be centered to the IR.
- **Grid use with cassette-less systems:** Anatomy thickness and kV range are deciding factors for whether a grid is to be used. With cassette-less systems it may be impractical and difficult to remove the grid. Therefore, the grid is commonly left in place even for smaller body parts measuring 10 cm or less. If the grid is left in place, it is important to ensure that the CR is centered to the grid for all projections.

Collimation and Shielding

A general rule for protective shielding states that it should be used whenever radiation-sensitive areas lie within or near the primary beam. Red bone marrow and gonadal tissues are two of the key radiation-sensitive regions. However, a good practice to follow, in addition to **close collimation** to the area of interest, is to use **gonadal shields** on youth and patients of childbearing age for **all** lower limb procedures. This provides assurance to the patient that he or she is being protected from unnecessary exposure.

Multiple Exposures per Imaging Plate

Multiple images can be placed on the same IP. When doing so, careful collimation and lead masking must be used to prevent pre-exposure or fogging of other images.

AP Toes

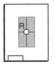

Alternative routine may include entire foot on AP toe projection for possible secondary trauma to other parts of foot (see AP foot).

- 18 × 24 cm C.W. (8 × 10″)
- Nongrid
- Lead masking with multiple exposures on same IR

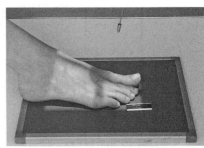

Fig. 4-1 AP 2nd digit, CR 10°-15° posteriorly.

Position

- Supine or seated on table with knee flexed, plantar surface of foot resting on IR
- Align long axis of affected toe(s) to portion of IR being exposed.

Central Ray:

- CR angled 10°-15° to calcaneus (⊥ to long axis of digits)
- CR centered to MTP joint(s) of interest

SID: 40-44″ (102-113 cm)

Collimation: Collimate on four sides to area of interest to include soft tissues.

kV Range:	Analog: 50-55 kV	Digital Systems: 55-60 kV

	cm	kV	mA	Time	mAs	SID	Exposure Indicator
S							
M							
L							

Bontrager Textbook, 8th ed, p. 226.

4

Lower Limb (Extremity)

AP Oblique Toes

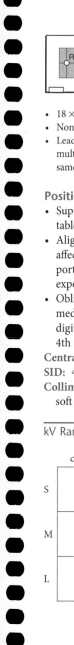

- 18 × 24 cm C.W. (8 × 10″)
- Nongrid
- Lead masking with multiple exposures on same IR

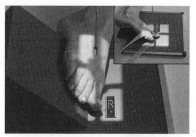

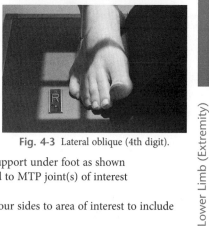

Fig. 4-2 Medial oblique (1st digit).

Position
- Supine or seated on table, foot resting on IR
- Align long axis of affected toe(s) to portion of IR being exposed
- Oblique foot 30°-45° medially for 1st to 3rd digits, and laterally for

Fig. 4-3 Lateral oblique (4th digit).

4th and 5th digits. Place support under foot as shown

Central Ray: CR ⊥, centered to MTP joint(s) of interest

SID: 40-44″ (102-113 cm)

Collimation: Collimate on four sides to area of interest to include soft tissues

kV Range:	Analog: 50-55 kV			Digital Systems: 55-60 kV		

	cm	kV	mA	Time	mAs	SID	Exposure Indicator
S							
M							
L							

Lower Limb (Extremity)

4

AP and AP Oblique Toes

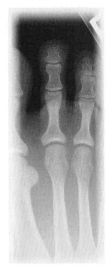

Fig. 4-4 AP toe.

Competency Check: _____
                  Technologist   Date

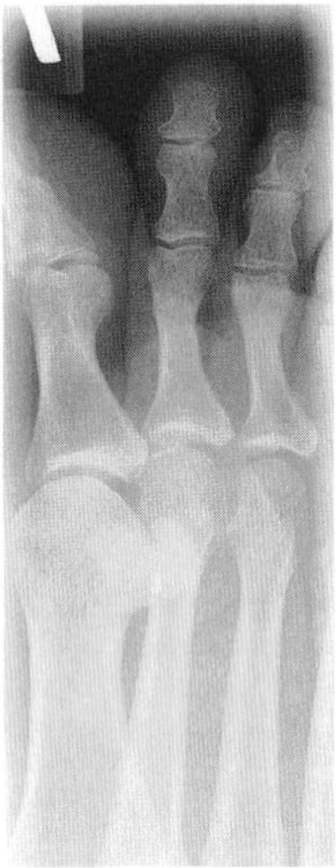

Fig. 4-5 AP oblique toe.

Competency Check: _____
                  Technologist   Date

Evaluation Criteria

Anatomy Demonstrated:

AP and AP Oblique
- Entire digit and minimum of $^1/_2$ of affected metatarsal

Position:
- **AP:** No overlap of surrounding digits and metatarsals; no rotation, equal concavity on both sides of shafts of phalanges and metatarsals
- **AP oblique:** Increased concavity on one side of phalangeal shaft

Exposure:
- Optimal density (brightness) and contrast; no motion
- Soft tissue and sharp cortical margins clearly demonstrated

Lateral Toes

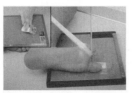

Fig. 4-6 Lateromedial (1st digit).

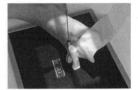

Fig. 4-7 Mediolateral (4th digit).

- 18×24 cm C.W. ($8 \times 10''$)
- Nongrid
- Lead masking with multiple exposures on same IR

Position

- Seated or recumbent on tabletop
- Carefully use tape and/or radiolucent gauze to help isolate unaffected digits as shown:

  1st to 3rd digits—lateromedial projection (1st digit down)

  4th to 5th digits—mediolateral projection (1st digit up)

Central Ray: CR ⊥, to IP joint for 1st digit, and to PIP joint for 2nd to 5th digits

SID: 40-44'' (102-113 cm)

Collimation: Collimate closely to digit of interest to include soft tissues

kV Range:	Analog: 50-55 kV				Digital Systems: 55-60 kV	
	cm	kV	mA	Time	mAs	SID	Exposure Indicator
S							
M							
L							

Lower Limb (Extremity)

Toes—Sesamoids
(Tangential Projection)

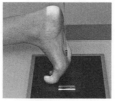

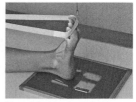

- 18 × 24 cm C.W. (8 × 10″)
- Nongrid
- Lead masking with multiple exposures on same IR

Fig. 4-8 Patient prone.

Fig. 4-9 Alternative supine position.

Position

- Patient prone with foot and great toe carefully dorsiflexed so the plantar surface forms a 15°-20° angle from vertical if possible (adjust CR angle as needed)

Alternative Supine Position: This may be a more tolerable position for patient to maintain if in great pain.

Central Ray: CR ⊥, or angled as needed to be 15°-20° from plantar surface of foot, centered to head of 1st metatarsal

SID: 40-44″ (102-113 cm)

Collimation: Collimate closely to area of interest; include distal 1st, 2nd, and 3rd metatarsals for possible sesamoids

	cm	kV	mA	Time	mAs	SID	Exposure Indicator
kV Range:		Analog: 50-55 kV			Digital Systems: 55-60 kV		
S							
M							
L							

Bontrager Textbook, 8th ed, p. 229.

Lower Limb (Extremity)

4

Evaluation Criteria

Anatomy Demonstrated:

- Entire digit, including proximal phalanx

Position:

- No superimposition of adjoining digits
- Proximal phalanx visualized through superimposed structures

Exposure:

- Contrast and density (brightness) sufficient to visualize soft tissue and bony portions; no motion

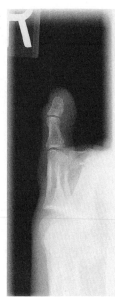

Fig. 4-10 Lateral second digit.

Competency Check: _____
                    Technologist Date

Tangential Projection
(Sesamoid Bones)

Evaluation Criteria

Anatomy Demonstrated:

- Sesamoid bones in profile

Position:

- No superimposition of sesamoids and 1st to 3rd distal metatarsals in profile

Exposure:

- Optimal density (brightness) and contrast; no motion
- Soft tissue and sharp cortical margins clearly demonstrated

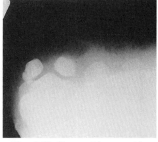

Fig. 4-11 Tangential sesamoids.

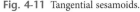

Competency Check: _____
                    Technologist Date

4

Lower Limb (Extremity)

107

AP Foot
(Dorsoplantar Projection)

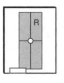

- 24 × 30 cm L.W. (10 × 12″)
- Nongrid
- Lead masking with multiple exposures on same IR

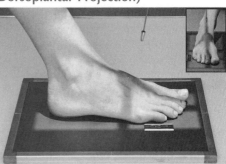

Fig. 4-12 AP foot, CR 10° posteriorly.

Position
- Supine or seated with plantar surface of foot flat on IR, aligned lengthwise to portion of IR being exposed
- Extend (plantar flex) foot by sliding foot and IR distally while keeping plantar surface flat on IR. (Support with sandbags to keep foot and IR from sliding farther.)

Central Ray: CR ⊥, to metatarsals, which is about 10° posteriorly (toward heel), centered to base of 3rd metatarsal

SID: 40-44″ (102-113 cm)

Collimation: Four sides to margins of foot

kV Range:	Analog: 60 ± 5 kV; or 70-75 kV and Reduced mAs	Digital Systems: 60-70 kV

	cm	kV	mA	Time	mAs	SID	Exposure Indicator
S							
M							
L							

Bontrager Textbook, 8th ed, p. 230.

AP Oblique Foot

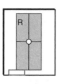

- 24 × 30 cm L.W. (10 × 12″)
- Nongrid
- Lead masking with multiple exposures on same IR

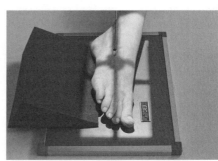

Fig. 4-13 30°-40° medial oblique.

Position

- Supine or seated with foot centered lengthwise to portion of IR being exposed
- Oblique foot 30°-40° medially, support with 45° radiolucent angle block and sandbags to prevent slippage
- **Note 1:** A higher arch requires nearer 45° oblique and a low arch "flat foot" nearer 30°.
- **Note 2**: A 30° lateral oblique projection will demonstrate the space between 1st and 2nd metatarsals and between 1st and 2nd cuneiforms.

Central Ray: CR ⊥, centered to base of 3rd metatarsal
SID: 40-44″ (102-113 cm)
Collimation: Four sides to margins of foot and distal ankle.

kV Range:	Analog: 60 ± 5 kV			Digital Systems: 60-70 kV		

	cm	kV	mA	Time	mAs	SID	Exposure Indicator
S							
M							
L							

Lower Limb (Extremity)

AP and AP (Medial) Oblique Foot

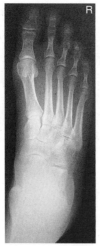

Fig. 4-14 AP foot.

Competency Check: _____
              Technologist   Date

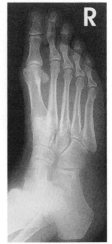

Fig. 4-15 Medial oblique foot.

Competency Check: _____
              Technologist   Date

Evaluation Criteria

Anatomy Demonstrated:

• **AP** and **AP medial oblique:** Tarsals, metatarsals, and phalanges

Position:

AP

• No rotation with tarsals superimposed

AP Medial Oblique

• 3rd to 5th metatarsals free of superimposition
• Cuboid clearly demonstrated; base of 5th metatarsal seen in profile

Exposure:

• Optimal density (brightness) and contrast; no motion
• Soft tissue and sharp bony trabeculation clearly demonstrated

Lateral Foot

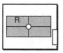

- 18 × 24 cm L.W. (8 × 10″) or
- 24 × 30 cm L.W. (10 × 12″) for large foot
- Nongrid

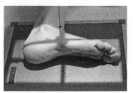

Fig. 4-16 Mediolateral foot.

Position
(Mediolateral)

- Recumbent, turned on affected side, knee flexed with unaffected leg behind to prevent overrotation
- Place support under affected knee and leg as needed to place plantar surface of foot perpendicular to IR for a true lateral.

Fig. 4-17 Lateromedial foot.

Lateromedial Projection: May be easier to achieve a true lateral if patient's condition allows this position.

Central Ray: CR ⊥, centered to area of base of third metatarsal

SID: 40-44″ (102-113 cm)

Collimation: Four sides to margins of foot and distal ankle

| kV Range: | Analog: 60 ± 5 kV | | | Digital Systems: 65-75 kV | | |

	cm	kV	mA	Time	mAs	SID	Exposure Indicator
S							
M							
L							

Lower Limb (Extremity)

4

Lateral Foot

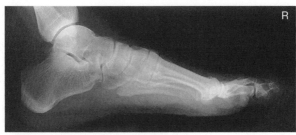

R

Fig. 4-18 Lateral foot.

Competency Check: _____

Technologist   Date

Evaluation Criteria

Anatomy Demonstrated:
- Entire foot with ≈1″ (2.5 cm) of distal tibia-fibula

Position:
- True lateral with tibiotalar joint open
- Distal metatarsals superimposed

Exposure:
- Optimal density (brightness) and contrast; no motion
- Soft tissue and sharp bony trabeculation clearly demonstrated

Lower Limb (Extremity)

Weight-Bearing Feet AP and Lateral

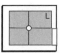

Lateral projection is most common for longitudinal arch (flat feet), AP demonstrates alignment of metatarsals and phalanges.

- 24 × 30 cm L.W. (10 × 12″); 35 × 43 cm C.W. (14 × 17″) for bilateral study
- Nongrid

Position

AP
Erect, weight evenly distributed on both feet, on one IR

Lateral
Erect, full weight on both feet, vertical IR between feet, standing on blocks, high enough from floor for horizontal CR (R and L feet taken for comparison)

Central Ray:

AP
CR 15° posteriorly, CR to level of base of 3rd metatarsal, midway between feet

Lateral
CR horizontal, to base of 5th metatarsal
SID: 40-44″ (102-113 cm)
Collimation: Collimate to outer skin margins of the feet

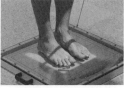

Fig. 4-19 AP—both feet CR 15° posteriorly.

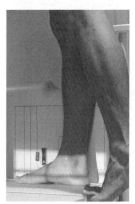

Fig. 4-20 Lateral—left foot.

4

Lower Limb (Extremity)

	kV Range:	Analog: **65 ± 5 kV**		Digital Systems: **60-70 kV**		

	cm	kV	mA	Time	mAs	SID	Exposure Indicator
S							
M							
L							

Bontrager Textbook, 8th ed., pp. 233 and 234.

Weight-Bearing AP and Lateral Foot

Evaluation Criteria
Anatomy Demonstrated:
- **AP:** Bilateral feet with soft tissue detail
- **Lateral:** Entire foot with 1" (2.5 cm) of distal tibia-fibula

Position:
- **AP:** Open tarsometatarsal joints; no rotation with approximately equal spacing of 2nd to 4th metatarsals
- **Lateral:** Dorsum to plantar surface demonstrated; heads of metatarsals superimposed

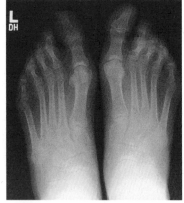

Fig. 4-21 AP weight-bearing foot.

Competency Check: _____
Technologist   Date

Exposure:
- Optimal density (brightness) and contrast
- Soft tissue and sharp bony trabeculation clearly demonstrated; no motion

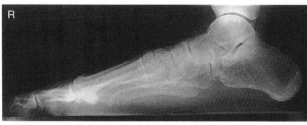

Fig. 4-22 Lateral weight-bearing foot.

Competency Check: _____
Technologist   Date

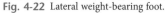

Lower Limb (Extremity)

Plantodorsal Calcaneus
(Axial Projection)

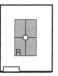

- 18 × 24 cm L.W. (8 × 10″)
- Nongrid (detail screens)
- Lead masking with multiple exposures on same IR

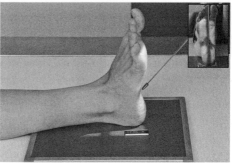

Fig. 4-23 CR 40° to long axis of foot.

Position

- Supine or seated, dorsiflex foot to as near vertical position as possible. If possible, have patient pull on gauze as shown. (This may be painful for patient to maintain, don't delay!)
- Center CR to part, with IR centered to projected CR.

Central Ray: CR 40° to long axis of plantar surface (may require more than 40° from vertical if foot is not dorsiflexed a full 90°)

- CR centered to base of 3rd metatarsal, to emerge just distal and inferior to ankle joint
- **Note**: Important to place the calcaneus on the lower aspect of the IR closest to the x-ray tube because of the severe CR angulation

SID: 40-44″ (102-113 cm)

Collimation: Collimate closely to region of calcaneus.

	cm	kV	mA	Time	mAs	SID	Exposure Indicator
kV Range:		Analog: 70 ± 5 kV			Digital Systems: 70-75 kV		
S							
M							
L							

Lower Limb (Extremity)

4

Lateral Calcaneus

- 18 × 24 cm
  L.W. (8 × 10")
- Nongrid
- Lead masking
  with multiple
  exposures on
  same IR

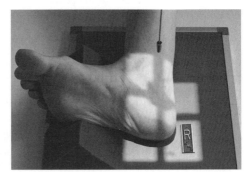

Fig. 4-24 Lateral calcaneus.

Position

- Recumbent, on affected side, knee flexed with unaffected limb behind, to prevent over-rotation
- Place support under knee and leg as needed for a true lateral
- Dorsiflex foot so the plantar surface is near 90° to leg if possible.

Central Ray: CR ⊥, to midcalcaneus, 1" (2.5 cm) inferior to medial malleolus

SID: 40-44" (102-113 cm)

Collimation: Four sides to area of calcaneus, include ankle joint at upper margin

kV Range:		Analog: **60 ± 5 kV**		Digital Systems: **60-70 kV**		

	cm	kV	mA	Time	mAs	SID	Exposure Indicator
S							
M							
L							

Bontrager Textbook, 8th ed., p. 236.

Plantodorsal (Axial) and Lateral Calcaneus

Evaluation Criteria
Anatomy Demonstrated:
- **Plantodorsal:** Entire calcaneus from tuberosity to talocalcaneal joint
- **Lateral:** Calcaneus in profile to distal tibia-fibula

Position:
- **Plantodorsal:** No rotation with sustentaculum tali in profile medially
- **Lateral:** Partial superimposed talus and open talocalcaneal joint

Exposure:
- Density and contrast (brightness) sufficient to faintly visualize distal fibula through talus; no motion
- Soft tissue and sharp bony trabeculation clearly demonstrated

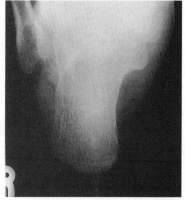

Fig. 4-25 Plantodorsal calcaneus.

Competency Check: _____
Technologist   Date

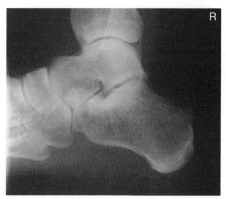

Fig. 4-26 Lateral calcaneus.

Competency Check: _____
Technologist   Date

4

Lower Limb (Extremity)

AP Ankle

- 24 × 30 cm L.W. (10 × 12″)
- Nongrid
- Lead masking with multiple exposures on same IR

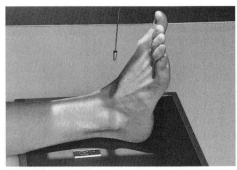

Fig. 4-27 AP ankle.

Position

- Supine or seated on table, leg extended, support under knee
- Align leg and ankle parallel to edge of IR.
- True AP, ensure no rotation, long axis of foot is vertical, parallel to CR (lateral malleolus will be about 15° more posterior than medial malleolus)

Central Ray: CR ⊥, to midway between malleoli

SID: 40-44″ (102-113 cm)

Collimation: Collimate to lateral skin margins; include proximal $^1/_2$ of metatarsals and distal tibia-fibula.

kV Range:	Analog: 60 ± 5 kV			Digital Systems: 60-70 kV			
	cm	kV	mA	Time	mAs	SID	Exposure Indicator
S							
M							
L							

Bontrager Textbook, 8th ed, p. 237.

AP Mortise Ankle

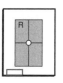

This is a frontal view of the entire ankle mortise and generally should not be a substitute for the routine AP or 45° oblique ankle.

- 24 × 30 cm L.W. (10 × 12″)
- Nongrid
- Lead masking with multiple exposures on same IR

Position

- Supine or seated on table, leg extended, support under knee
- Rotate leg and long axis of foot internally 15°-20° so **intermalleolar line is parallel to tabletop.**

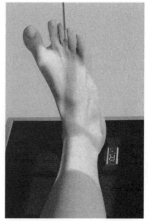

Fig. 4-28 AP, to visualize entire ankle mortise (15°-20° medial oblique).

Central Ray: CR ⊥, to midway between malleoli

SID: 40-44″ (102-113 cm)

Collimation: Collimate to ankle region. Include distal tibia-fibula and proximal metatarsals in collimation field.

Note: The base of the fifth metatarsal is a common fracture site and may be demonstrated in this projection.

kV Range:	Analog: 60 ± 5 kV	Digital Systems: 60-70 kV

	cm	kV	mA	Time	mAs	SID	Exposure Indicator
S							
M							
L							

4

Lower Limb (Extremity)

AP Oblique Ankle

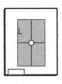

- 24 × 30 cm L.W. (10 × 12″)
- Nongrid
- Lead masking with multiple exposures on same IR

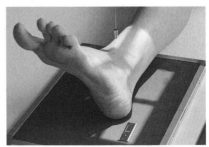

Fig. 4-29 45° medial oblique ankle.

Position

- Supine or seated, leg extended, support under knee
- Rotate leg and foot 45° internally (long axis of foot is 45° to IR).

Central Ray: CR ⊥, to midway between the malleoli

SID: 40-44″ (102-113 cm)

Collimation: Collimate to ankle region, include proximal metatarsals and distal tibia-fibula.

Note: The base of 5th metatarsal is a common fracture site and may be visualized on oblique ankle projections.

kV Range: Analog: 60 ± 5 kV   Digital Systems: 60-70 kV

	cm	kV	mA	Time	mAs	SID	Exposure Indicator
S							
M							
L							

Bontrager Textbook, 8th ed, p. 239.

AP, AP Mortise, and 45° Oblique Ankle

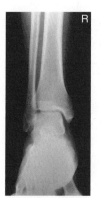

Fig. 4-30 AP ankle.

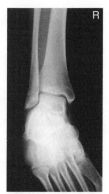

Fig. 4-31 AP mortise ankle.

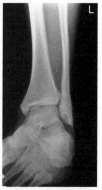

Fig. 4-32 45° oblique.

Competency _____
Check: Technologist Date

Evaluation Criteria

Anatomy Demonstrated:
- **AP:** Distal $^{1}/_{3}$ tibia-fibula, talus, and proximal metatarsals
- **AP mortise:** Entire ankle mortise with distal $^{1}/_{3}$ tibia-fibula and base of 5th metatarsal; equal distance throughout the tibiotalar joint
- **AP 45° oblique:** Distal $^{1}/_{3}$ tibia-fibula, talus, calcaneus, and base of 5th metatarsal

Position:
- **AP:** No rotation with superior-medial joint surfaces open.
- **AP mortise:** Open lateral, superior, and medial joint surfaces; malleoli in profile
- **AP 45° oblique:** Open distal tibiofibular joint, talus, and medial malleolus open with no or only minimal overlap.

Exposure:
- Density and contrast (brightness) sufficient to faintly visualize distal fibula through talus; no motion
- Soft tissue and sharp bony trabeculation clearly demonstrated

Lower Limb (Extremity)

4

121

Lateral Ankle

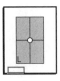

- 24 × 30 cm L.W. (10 × 12")
- Nongrid (detail screens)
- Lead masking with multiple exposures on same IR

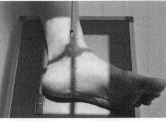

Fig. 4-33 Mediolateral ankle.

Position

- Recumbent, affected side down, affected knee partially flexed
- Dorsiflex foot 90° to leg if patient can tolerate.
- Place support under knee as needed for true lateral of foot and ankle.

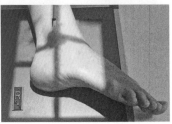

Fig. 4-34 Lateromedial ankle.

Central Ray: CR ⊥, to medial malleolus

Note: May also be taken as a lateromedial projection if patient condition allows, may be easier to achieve a true lateral.

SID: 40-44" (102-113 cm)

Collimation: Four sides to ankle region. Include distal tibia-fibula and proximal metatarsals.

kV Range:	Analog: 60 ± 5 kV				Digital Systems: 60-70 kV	
	cm	kV	mA	Time	mAs	SID	Exposure Indicator
S							
M							
L							

Bontrager Textbook, 8th ed, p. 240.

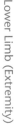

4

Lower Limb (Extremity)

Lateral Ankle

Evaluation Criteria
Anatomy Demonstrated:
- Distal $^1/_3$ of tibia-fibula with lateral view of tarsals and base of 5th metatarsal

Position:
- True lateral with no rotation, distal fibula superimposed **over posterior half of tibia**
- Tibiotalar joint open

Exposure:
- Density and contrast (brightness) sufficient to faintly visualize distal fibula through talus; no motion
- Soft tissue and sharp bony trabeculation clearly demonstrated

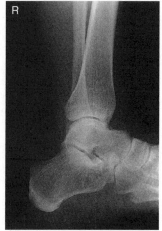

Fig. 4-35 Lateral ankle.

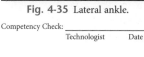

Competency Check: _____
　　　　　　　　　Technologist　　Date

4

AP Ankle—Stress Views
(Inversion and Eversion Positions)

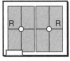

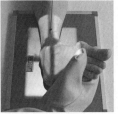

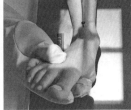

Fig. 4-36 Inversion stress.   **Fig. 4-37** Eversion stress.

Warning: Stress must be applied very carefully, either by a long gauze held by patient or handheld by qualified person wearing lead gloves and apron (may require injection of local anesthetic by a physician).

- 24 × 30 cm L.W. (10 × 12″) or 35 × 43 cm C.W. (14 × 17″)
- Nongrid
- Lead masking with multiple exposures on same IR

Position
- Supine or seated on table, leg extended
- Without rotating leg or ankle (true AP), stress is applied to ankle joint by first turning plantar surface of foot inward (inversion stress), then outward (eversion stress).

Central Ray: CR ⊥, to midway between malleoli
SID: 40-44″ (102-113 cm)
Collimation: Collimate to lateral skin margins, including proximal metatarsals and distal tibia-fibula.

	cm	kV	mA	Time	mAs	SID	Exposure Indicator
kV Range:	Analog: 60 ± 5 kV			Digital Systems: 60-70 kV			
S							
M							
L							

Bontrager Textbook, 8th ed, p. 241.

AP Leg (Tibia-Fibula)

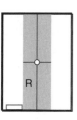

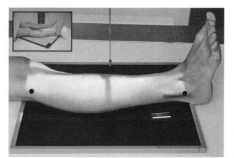

Fig. 4-38 AP leg.

- 35 × 43 cm L.W.
  (14 × 17″) diagonal
  only if needed to
  include both ankle
  and knee joints.
- Nongrid
- Knee at cathode end to utilize anode heel effect

Position

- Supine, leg extended, ensure no rotation of knee, leg, or ankle
- Include ≈3 cm (1-1.5″) minimum beyond knee and ankle joints,
  considering divergent rays

Central Ray: CR ⊥, to midshaft of leg (to mid-IR)

SID: Minimum SID of 40″ (102 cm); may increase to 44-48″
(112-123 cm)

Collimation: On four sides, to include knee and ankle joints

4

Lower Limb (Extremity)

kV Range:		Analog: 70 ± 5 kV			Digital Systems: 70-80 kV	

	cm	kV	mA	Time	mAs	SID	Exposure Indicator
S							
M							
L							

Lethal Leg (Tibia-Fibula)

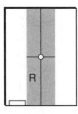

- 35 × 43 cm L.W. (14 × 17″) diagonal if needed to include both joints
- Nongrid

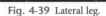

Fig. 4-39 Lateral leg.

- Knee at cathode end (to utilize anode heel effect)

Position

- Recumbent, affected side down
- Place unaffected limb behind patient to prevent over-rotation.
- Place support under distal portion of affected foot as needed to ensure a true lateral position of foot, ankle, and knee.
- Include ≈3 cm (1-1.5″) minimum beyond knee and ankle joints considering divergent rays

Central Ray: CR ⊥, to midshaft of leg (to mid-IR)

SID: Minimum SID of 40″ (102 cm); may increase to 44-48″ (112-123 cm)

Collimation: On four sides, to include knee and ankle joints

kV Range:	Analog: 70 ± 5 kV			Digital Systems: 70-80 kV		

	cm	kV	mA	Time	mAs	SID	Exposure Indicator
S							
M							
L							

Bontrager Textbook, 8th ed, p. 243.

AP and Lateral Leg (Tibia-Fibula)

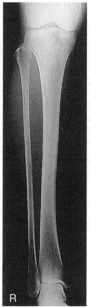

Fig. 4-40 AP lower leg.

Competency Check: _____
                        Technologist   Date

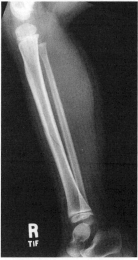

Fig. 4-41 Lateral lower leg.

Competency Check: _____
                        Technologist   Date

Evaluation Criteria

Anatomy Demonstrated:

- **AP:** Entire tibia-fibula with ankle and knee joints
- **Lateral:** Entire tibia-fibula with ankle and knee joints

Position:

- **AP:** No rotation, with femoral and tibial condyles in profile
- Slight overlap at both proximal and distal tibiofibular joints
- **Lateral:** Tibial tuberosity in profile
- Distal fibula overlaps posterior portion of tibia

Exposure:

- Near equal density (brightness) and contrast; no motion
- Soft tissue and sharp bony trabeculation clearly demonstrated

AP Knee

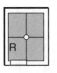

- 24 × 30 cm L.W. (10 × 12″)
- Grid >10 cm
- IR <10 cm

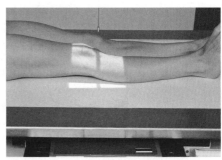

Fig. 4-42 AP knee (CR ⊥, to film for average patient).

Position
- Supine, or seated on table, with leg extended and centered to CR and midline of table or IR
- Rotate leg slightly inward as needed to place knee and leg into a true AP. Center IR to CR.

Central Ray: CR centered to 1.25 cm ($^1/_2$″) distal to apex of patella

CR Parallel to Articular Facets (Tibial Plateau): Measure distance from ASIS to TT to determine CR angle.
- Thin thighs and buttocks (<19 cm ASIS to TT), **3°-5° caudad**
- Average thighs and buttocks (19-24 cm), **0°, ⊥ IR**
- Thick thighs and buttocks (>24 cm), **3°-5° cephalad**

SID: 40-44″ (102-113 cm)

Collimation: Sides to skin borders, ends to IR borders

---

kV Range:	Analog: 65 ± 5 kV			Digital Systems: 70-85 kV		
	cm	kV	mA	Time	mAs	SID	Exposure Indicator
S							
M							
L							

Bontrager Textbook, 8th ed, p. 244.

4

Lower Limb (Extremity)

AP Oblique Knee

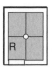

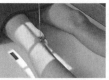

Fig. 4-43 45° medial oblique.

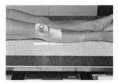

Fig. 4-44 45° lateral oblique.

Medial oblique: Demonstrates fibular head and neck unobscured. (Lateral oblique may also be taken.)
- 24 × 30 cm L.W. (10 × 12″)
- Grid >10 cm
- IR <10 cm

Position
- Supine, leg extended and centered to CR and midline of table
- Rotate entire leg, including knee, ankle, and foot, internally 45° for medial oblique, and 45° externally for external oblique
- Center IR to CR.

Central Ray:
- CR ⊥, to IR on average patient (see AP Knee)
- CR to mid-joint space (1.25 cm or $^1/_2$″ inferior to patella)

SID: 40-44″ (102-113 cm)

Collimation: Sides to skin borders, ends to IR borders

| | kV Range: | Analog: **65 ± 5 kV** | | Digital Systems: **70-85 kV** |

	cm	kV	mA	Time	mAs	SID	Exposure Indicator
S							
M							
L							

Lower Limb (Extremity)

AP and AP Medial and Lateral Oblique Knee

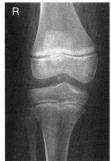
Fig. 4-45 AP knee.

Competency
Check: _____
Technologist   Date

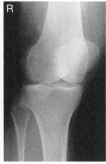
Fig. 4-46 AP medial oblique.

Competency _____
Check: Technologist   Date

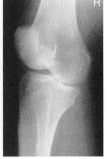
Fig. 4-47 AP lateral oblique.

Competency _____
Check: Technologist   Date

Evaluation Criteria

Anatomy Demonstrated:

- **AP:** Open femorotibial joint space
- **AP medial oblique:** Open proximal tibiofibular joint; femoral and tibial lateral condyles in profile
- **AP lateral oblique:** Medial condyles in profile

Position:

- **AP:** No rotation evident by symmetric appearance of femoral and tibial condyles
- **AP medial oblique:** Proximal tibiofibular joint open; tibial lateral condyles demonstrated
- **AP lateral oblique:** Medial condyles of femur and tibia are in profile; proximal tibia and fibula are superimposed

Exposure:

- Optimal density (brightness) and contrast; outline of patella through distal femur; no motion
- Soft tissue and sharp bony trabeculation clearly demonstrated

Lower Limb (Extremity)

Lateral Knee

- 24 × 30 cm L.W. (10 × 12″)
- Grid >10 cm
- IR <10 cm

Position

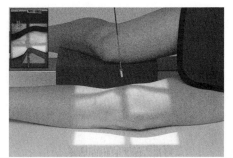

Fig. 4-48 Mediolateral knee, CR 5° cephalad.

- Patient on affected side, knee flexed ≈20°, centered to CR and midline of table or IR
- Unaffected leg and knee placed behind to prevent over-rotation
- Place support under affected ankle and foot if needed and adjust body rotation as required for a true lateral of knee.
- Center IR to CR.

Central Ray:
- CR 5°-7° cephalad
- CR centered to ≈2.5 cm (1″) distal to medial epicondyle

SID: 40-44″ (102-113 cm)

Collimation: Sides to skin borders, ends to borders of IR

	kV Range:	Analog: 65 ± 5 kV			Digital Systems: 70-85 kV		
	cm	kV	mA	Time	mAs	SID	Exposure Indicator
S							
M							
L							

Lower Limb (Extremity)

4

Lateral Knee

Evaluation Criteria
Anatomy Demonstrated:
- Distal femur, proximal tibia-fibula, and patella in lateral profile
- Femoropatellar and knee joints open

Position:
- True lateral with no rotation; femoral condyles superimposed
- Patella in profile and femoropatellar joint open

Exposure:
- Optimal density (brightness) and contrast; no motion
- Soft tissue (fat pads) and sharp bony trabeculation clearly demonstrated

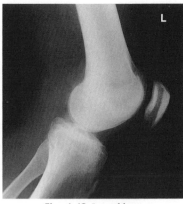

Fig. 4-49 Lateral knee.

Competency Check: _____

Technologist   Date

Knees—AP or PA Weight-Bearing

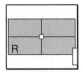

- 35 × 43 cm C.W. (14 × 17″)
- Grid

Position

AP:

- Erect, standing on step stool or footboard as needed (high enough to get x-ray tube low for horizontal beam)

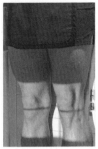

Fig. 4-50 AP weight-bearing—bilateral, CR ⊥ to IR.

- Feet straight ahead, knees straight, weight distributed evenly on both feet. Have patient hold onto table handles for support.

Alternative PA: Patient facing the table or IR holder, with knees against table or vertical IR holder, knees flexed ≈20°

Central Ray: CR to midpoint between knee joints, at level of ≈1.25 cm ($^1/_2$″) distal to apex of patellae

AP: CR horizontal, ⊥ to IR on average patient (see AP Knee)

PA: CR 10° caudad (if knees are flexed ≈20°)

SID: 40-44″ (102-113 cm)

Collimation: To bilateral knee joint region

Lower Limb (Extremity)

kV Range:	Analog: 70 ± 5 kV			Digital Systems: 70-85 kV			
	cm	kV	mA	Time	mAs	SID	Exposure Indicator
S							
M							
L							

PA Axial Weight-Bearing Bilateral Knees
(Rosenberg Method)

- 35 × 43 cm C.W.
  (14 × 17″)
- Grid

Position
- Patient erect PA
- Weight evenly distributed
- Knees flexed to 45°

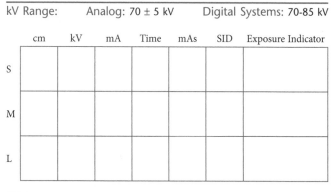

Fig. 4-51 PA axial weight-bearing—CR 10° caudad.

Fig. 4-52 Rosenberg method.

Central Ray: 10° caudad to mid-knee joints—¹/₂″ (1.25 cm) below apex of patella.

SID: 40-44″ (102-113 cm)

Collimation: Bilateral knee joint region, including distal femora and proximal tibia

	cm	kV	mA	Time	mAs	SID	Exposure Indicator
kV Range:		Analog: 70 ± 5 kV			Digital Systems: 70-85 kV		
S							
M							
L							

Bontrager Textbook, 8th ed, p. 249.

PA Axial Weight-Bearing Bilateral Knees
(Rosenberg Method)

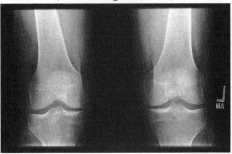

Fig. 4-53 PA axial weight-bearing knees.

Competency Check: _____

Technologist   Date

Evaluation Criteria

Anatomy Demonstrated:
- Distal femur, proximal tibia and fibula, femorotibial joint spaces, and intercondylar fossa

Position:
- **No rotation** of both knees evident by symmetric appearance
- Articular facets in profile

Exposure:
- Optimal density (brightness) and contrast; no motion
- Soft tissue and sharp bony trabeculation clearly demonstrated

Lower Limb (Extremity)

135

Knee for Intercondylar Fossa
Camp Coventry and Holmblad Methods (Tunnel View)

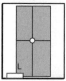

- 18 × 24 cm L.W. (8 × 10″)
- Grid

Camp Coventry:
Position:
- Prone, knee flexed 40°-50°, large support under ankle
- Knee centered to CR
- IR centered to projected CR

Central Ray: CR 40°-50° caudad (⊥ to lower leg), centered to knee joint, to emerge at distal margin of patella
SID: 40-44″ (102-113 cm)
Collimation: Four sides to area of interest

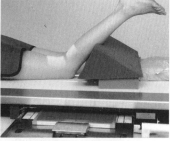

Fig. 4-54 PA axial projection (Camp Coventry).

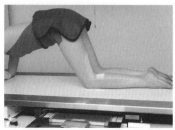

Fig. 4-55 Alternative Holmblad method:
– Patient kneeling, leans forward 20°-30°
– CR ⊥ to IR

4

Lower Limb (Extremity)

	cm	kV	mA	Time	mAs	SID	Exposure Indicator
kV Range:	Analog: 70 ± 5 kV			Digital Systems: 70-85 kV			
S							
M							
L							

Bontrager Textbook, 8th ed, pp. 251 and 252.

PA Patella

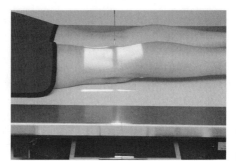

- 18 × 24 cm L.W.
  (8 × 10″)
- Grid

Position
- Prone, knee centered to CR and midline of table or IR

Fig. 4-56 PA patella.

- If patella area is painful, place pad under thigh and leg to prevent direct pressure on patella.
- Rotate anterior knee approximately 5° internally or as needed to place an imaginary line between the epicondyles parallel to the plane of the IR.
- Center IR to CR.

Central Ray: CR ⊥, centered to central patella region (at midpopliteal crease)

SID: 40-44″ (102-113 cm)

Collimation: To area of patella and knee joint

kV Range:		Analog: 75 ± 5 kV (Increase 6 kV from PA Knee)				Digital Systems: 70-85 kV

	cm	kV	mA	Time	mAs	SID	Exposure Indicator
S							
M							
L							

Bontrager Textbook, 8th ed, p. 254.

Lateral Patella

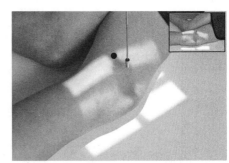

- 18 × 24 cm L.W. (8 × 10″)
- Nongrid (detail screens—may use grid on large patient)

Fig. 4-57 Lateral patella.

Position
- Recumbent on affected side, opposite knee, and leg behind to prevent over-rotation
- Flex knee only 5°-10° to prevent separation of fractured fragments if present.
- Patellofemoral joint area centered to CR and midline of IR.

Central Ray: CR ⊥, centered to mid-patellofemoral joint space
SID: 40-44″ (102-113 cm)
Collimation: To area of knee joint, patella, and patellofemoral joint

kV Range:		Analog: 70 ± 6 kV			Digital Systems: 70-80 kV		
	cm	kV	mA	Time	mAs	SID	Exposure Indicator
S							
M							
L							

Bontrager Textbook, 8th ed, p. 255.

Intercondylar Fossa, PA and Lateral Patella

Evaluation Criteria

Anatomy Demonstrated:

- **PA axial:** Intercondylar fossa shown in profile
- **PA:** Knee joint and patella outline through distal femur
- **Lateral:** Lateral patella in profile

Position:

- **PA axial:** No rotation evidenced by symmetric femoral condyles and intercondylar eminence centered under intercondylar fossa
- **PA:** No rotation, femoral condyles appear symmetric; patella appears centered to femur
- **Lateral:** Patella in profile and femoropatellar joint open

Exposure:

- Optimal density (brightness) and contrast; no motion
- Sharp bony trabeculation clearly demonstrated

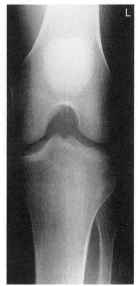

Fig. 4-58 PA axial—intercondylar fossa projection.

Competency Check: _____
Technologist   Date

4

Lower Limb (Extremity)

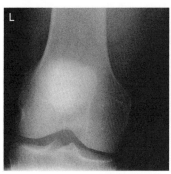

Fig. 4-59 PA patella.

Competency Check: _____
Technologist   Date

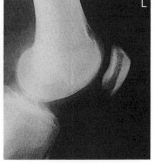

Fig. 4-60 Lateral patella.

Competency Check: _____
Technologist   Date

Patella—Tangential Projection
(Merchant Bilateral Method)

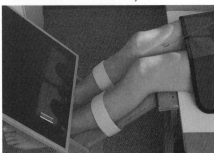

Fig. 4-61 Bilateral tangential.

- 24 × 30 cm C.W. (10 × 12″) or 35 × 43 cm (14 × 17″) C.W. for large knees
- Nongrid
- Adjustable leg and IR-holding device required

Position
- Supine with knees flexed 45° on leg supports (important for patient to be comfortable with legs totally relaxed to prevent patellae from being drawn into intercondylar sulcus)
- Place IR on supports against legs about 30 cm (12″) distal to patellae, perpendicular to CR.
- Internally rotate both legs as needed to center patellae to midfemora.

Central Ray: CR 30° from horizontal (30° from long axis of femora)
- CR to midpoint between patellae at patellofemoral joints

SID: 48-72″ (123-183 cm) greater SID reduces magnification

Collimation: To bilateral patellae and patellofemoral joints

kV Range:	Analog: 65 ± 5 kV			Digital Systems: 70-80 kV		
	cm	kV	mA	Time	mAs	SID	Exposure Indicator
S							
M							
L							

Bontrager Textbook, 8th ed, p. 256.

Patella—Tangential Projection
(Settegast and Hughston Methods)

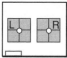

Generally taken bilaterally for comparison purposes.

- 24 × 30 cm C.W. (10 × 12″)
- Nongrid
- Lead masking with multiple exposures on same IR

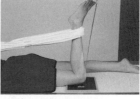

Fig. 4-62 Settegast:
– Knee flexed 90°
– CR 15°-20° to leg

Position

- Prone, knee flexed as shown
- Use long gauze or tape for patient to hold leg in position; for Hughston method, may support foot on collimator, use pad

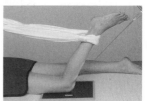

Fig. 4-63 Hughston:
– Knee flexed 45°
– CR 10°-15° to leg
Warning: Possible **hot** collimator, use pad.

Central Ray: CR centered to patellofemoral joint space

Settegast: CR 15°-20° cephalad to long axis of leg (knee flexed 90°)

Hughston: CR 15°-20° cephalad to long axis of leg (knee flexed 45°) (recommended method)

SID: 40-48″ (102-123 cm)

Collimate: Closely to patella region

4

Lower Limb (Extremity)

kV Range:	Analog: 65 ± 5 kV			Digital Systems: 70-80 kV			
	cm	kV	mA	Time	mAs	SID	Exposure Indicator
S							
M							
L							

Patella—Superoinferior Sitting Tangential
(Hobbs Modification)

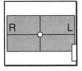

Generally taken bilaterally for comparison purposes

- 35 × 43 cm C.W. (14 × 17″) or 18 × 24 cm (8 × 10″), C.W. (unilateral)
- Nongrid

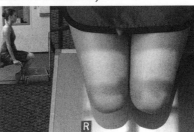

Fig. 4-64 Tangential superoinferior (Hobbs modification).

Position

- Patient seated
- Knees flexed with feet placed under chair
- IR placed on footstool

Central Ray: Perpendicular to IR centered to midway between femoropatellar joints

SID: 48-50″ (123-128 cm)

Collimation: Bilateral knee joint region, distal femora, and patella

kV Range:	Analog: 65 ± 5 kV			Digital Systems: 70-80 kV		
	cm	kV	mA	Time	mAs	SID	Exposure Indicator
S							
M							
L							

Bontrager Textbook, 8th ed, p. 258.

Tangential Bilateral Patella
(Hobbs Modification)

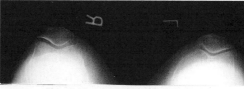

Fig. 4-65 Tangential sitting method.

Competency Check: _____
                    Technologist   Date

Evaluation Criteria
Anatomy Demonstrated:
- Tangential view of patella
- Femoropatellar knee joint

Position:
- Separation of patella and intercondylar sulcus
- Femoropatellar joint open

Exposure:
- Optimal density (brightness) and contrast; no motion
- Soft tissue and sharp bony trabeculation clearly demonstrated

Lower Limb (Extremity)

Pediatric AP Lower Limb

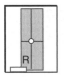

- Size determined by patient size
- Nongrid (detail screen)

Note: If foot is specific area of interest, AP and lateral projections of foot only may be required.

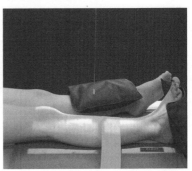

Fig. 4-66 AP lower limb.

Position—Shield Gonads

- Supine, include entire limb, shield over pelvic area
- A second IR of pelvis and/or proximal femur may be required (see Chapter 16 in the text)
- Immobilize arms and unaffected leg with sandbags.
- Use parental assistance only if necessary; provide lead gloves and apron.

Central Ray: CR ⊥, centered to midlimb (mid-IR)

SID: 40-44″ (102-113 cm)

Collimation: Four sides to area of interest

	cm	kV	mA	Time	mAs	SID	Exposure Indicator
S							
M							
L							

kV Range: Analog and Digital Systems: 55-60 kV

Bontrager Textbook, 8th ed, p. 637.

Pediatric Lateral Lower Limb

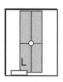

- Size determined by patient size
- Nongrid (detail screen)

Note: If foot is specific area of interest, AP and lateral projections of foot only may also be required.

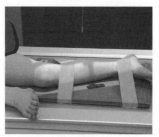

Fig. 4-67 Lateral lower limb (see *Note*).

Position—Shield Gonads

- Semisupine, include entire limb, shield over pelvic area
- Immobilize arms and unaffected leg with sandbags as needed
- Abduct (frog leg) affected limb into lateral position, immobilize with tape or compression band. (Do not attempt with hip trauma or hip disease.)
- If parental assistance is necessary, provide lead gloves and apron

Central Ray: CR ⊥, centered to midlimb (mid-IR)

SID: 40″ (102 cm)

Collimation: Four sides to area of interest

kV Range:	Analog: 55-70 kV			Digital Systems: 55-60 kV		
	cm	kV	mA	Time	mAs	SID	Exposure Indicator
S							
M							
L							

Pediatric—AP and Lateral Foot
(Congenital Clubfoot—Kite Method)

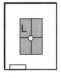

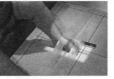

Fig. 4-68 AP foot.

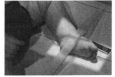

Fig. 4-69 Mediolateral foot.

- 18 × 24 cm L.W. (8 × 10")
- Nongrid (detail screens)

Note: With **Kite method,** no attempt is made to straighten foot when placing on IR. The foot is held or immobilized for a frontal and side view (AP and lateral projections) 90° from each other. Both feet generally are taken for comparison.

Position
- **AP:** Elevate patient on support, flex knee, foot on IR
- **Lateral:** Patient and/or leg on side, affected side down, use tape or compression band

Central Ray:
- **AP:** CR ⊥, to IR, directed to midtarsals (Kite suggests no angle)
- **Lateral:** CR ⊥, centered to proximal metatarsal area

SID: 40-44" (102-113 cm)

Collimation: Closely on four sides to area of foot

	cm	kV	mA	Time	mAs	SID	Exposure Indicator
S							
M							
L							

kV Range: Analog: 55-70 kV   Digital Systems: 60-70 kV

Bontrager Textbook, 8th ed, p. 638.

4

Lower Limb (Extremity)

Chapter 5

Femur and Pelvic Girdle

(R) Routine, (S) Special

5

Femur and Pelvic Girdle

Femur and Pelvic Girdle

Radiation Protection

Male: Gonadal shields should be used on pelvis and hip procedures for **all** male children and adults of childbearing age. Contact shields should be placed over the testes with the upper edge of the shield placed at the inferior margin of the symphysis pubis.

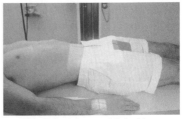

Fig. 5-1 Male gonadal shielding.

Female: For AP and "frog-leg" laterals of the hips, specially shaped ovarian shields can be carefully placed over the area of the ovaries without obscuring essential anatomy as shown. This should be done on all female children and adults of childbearing age. These ovarian shields, however, may obscure essential

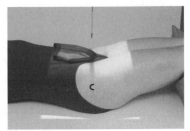

Fig. 5-2 Female ovarian shielding (superior borders at or slightly above level of ASISs and lower border just above pubis).

anatomy on certain pelvic examinations. Departmental policy regarding shielding and kV range to be used should be determined.

kV Range: A higher kV range (90 ± 5) with lower mAs may be used for examinations of the hips and pelvis of adults to reduce the total radiation dose to the patient.

Close collimation to the area of interest is important for all procedures, including the hips and pelvis, even with gonadal shields. (See Appendix A for further explanation.)

Location of Femoral Head and Neck

First Method: Location of the femoral head and neck regions can be accurately determined by first drawing an imaginary line between two landmarks, the **ASIS** and the **symphysis pubis**. The midpoint of this line is determined, from which a perpendicular imaginary line is drawn to locate the head and/or neck. The femoral head (A) is approximately 1.5″ (4 cm) down on this line. The midfemoral neck (B) is approximately 2.5″ (6-7 cm) down, as shown in the photo below.

Second Method: A second method for locating the femoral neck (B) is ≈1-2″ (3-5 cm) medial to the ASIS at the level of the proximal or upper margin of the symphysis pubis, which is 3-4″ (8-10 cm) distal to the ASIS.

Method one:
Head-1.5″
(4 cm)
Neck-2.5″
(6-7 cm)

Method two:
1-2″
(3-5 cm)

3-4″
(8-10 cm)

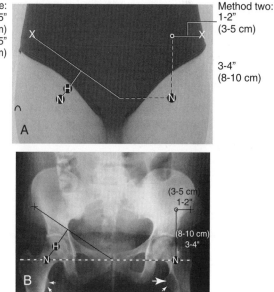

(3-5 cm)
1-2″

(8-10 cm)
3-4″

Fig. 5-3 **A,** Femoral head. **B,** Femoral neck.

AP Femur

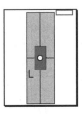

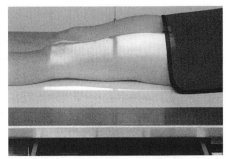

- 35 × 43 cm L.W. (14 × 17″)
- Grid
- Hip at cathode end (anode heel effect)

Fig. 5-4 AP, midfemur and distal femur.

Note: For adults, a second smaller IR of either the hip or the knee should be taken on trauma patients to demonstrate both knee and hip joints to rule out possible fractures.

Position
- Supine, femur centered to midline of table or grid IR
- Rotate entire lower limb internally ≈5° for AP of midfemur and distal femur, and 15° internally for true AP to include hip.
- Lower border of IR ≈5 cm (2″) below knee to include knee joint adequately (see AP Unilateral Hip for proximal femur, p. 156).
- **Shield gonads** for both male and female

Central Ray: CR ⊥, to mid-IR

SID: 40-44″ (102-113 cm)

Collimation: Long, narrow collimation to femur area

kV Range:	Analog: 75 ± 5 kV			Digital Systems: 75-85 kV		

	cm	kV	mA	Time	mAs	SID	Exposure Indicator
S							
M							
L							

Bontrager Textbook, 8th ed, p. 274.

Femur and Pelvic Girdle

5

Lateral Femur

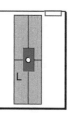

Warning: Take horizontal beam lateral if fracture is suspected.

- 35 × 43 cm L.W. (14 × 17″)
- Grid
- Hip at cathode end (anode heel effect)

Note: For adults, take a second smaller IR of lateral hip or lateral knee if both joints are areas of interest.

Position

- Lateral recumbent, with unaffected leg placed behind to prevent over-rotation
- Include sufficient amount of either knee or hip at one end of IR.
- Shield gonads as possible.

Central Ray: CR ⊥, to mid-IR
SID: 40-44″ (102-113 cm)
Collimation: Long, narrow collimation to femur area

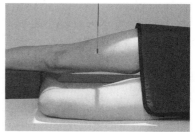

Fig. 5-5 Lateral, midfemur, and distal femur.

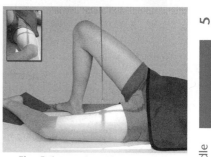

Fig. 5-6 Lateral, midfemur, and proximal femur.

| kV Range: | Analog: 75 ± 5 kV | | | Digital Systems: 75-85 kV | | |

	cm	kV	mA	Time	mAs	SID	Exposure Indicator
S							
M							
L							

AP and Lateral Midfemur and Distal Femur

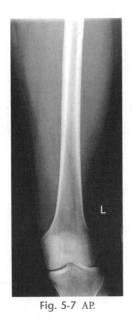

Fig. 5-7 AP.

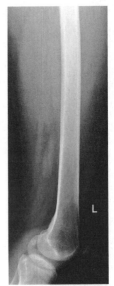

Fig. 5-8 Lateral.

Competency Check: _____
                    Technologist   Date

Competency Check: _____
                    Technologist   Date

Evaluation Criteria
Anatomy Demonstrated:
AP and Lateral
- Distal $^2/_3$ of femur, including knee joint

Position:
AP
- No rotation, femoral and tibial condyles appear symmetric in size and shape

Lateral
- True lateral, femoral condyles appear superimposed

Exposure:
AP and Lateral
- Optimal density and contrast
- Sharp borders and trabecular markings; no motion

152

Horizontal Beam Lateral Femur
(Trauma Midfemur and Distal Femur)

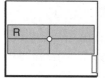

- 35 × 43 cm L.W. (14 × 17″)
- Portable grid

Note: For proximal femur injuries, take axiolateral (Danelius-Miller method) hip.

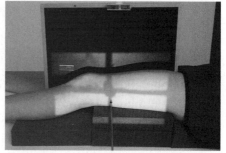

Fig. 5-9 Horizontal beam trauma projection (midfemur and distal femur).

Position

- Without moving trauma patient from the supine position, gently lift injured leg and place support under knee and leg.
- Place vertical IR between legs, as far superiorly as possible, but include knee distally. Use tape to hold grid IR in position.
- **Shield gonads** for both male and female.

Central Ray: CR horizontal beam, ⊥ to mid-IR

SID: 40-44″ (102-113 cm)

Collimation: Four sides to area of interest

kV Range:　　Analog: **75 ± 5 kV**　　Digital Systems: **75-80 kV**

	cm	kV	mA	Time	mAs	SID	Exposure Indicator
S							
M							
L							

Femur and Pelvic Girdle

AP Bilateral Hips

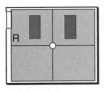

Warning: Do not attempt to rotate leg if fracture is suspected. Take "as is" bilateral hips for comparison purposes.

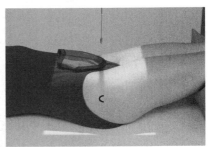

Fig. 5-10 AP bilateral hips.

Note: For AP pelvis centering, see p. 291 in text.

- 35 × 43 cm C.W. (14 × 17")
- Grid

Position

- Supine, aligned and centered to CR and IR, both legs extended and equally rotated internally 15°-20° (see warning above)
- Ensure no rotation of pelvis (bilateral ASISs the same distances from tabletop). Support under knees for patient comfort.
- Center IR to CR. **Shield gonads** (males and females).

Central Ray: CR ⊥, to midpoint between femoral heads (which is about 2 cm or 1" superior to symphysis pubis)

SID: 40-44" (102-113 cm)

Collimation: To pelvic and hip borders

Respiration: Suspend during exposure.

---

kV Range:		Analog: 80 ± 5 kV			Digital Systems: 80-85 kV	
	cm	kV	mA	Time	mAs	SID	Exposure Indicator
S							
M							
L							

Bontrager Textbook, 8th ed, p. 277.

Femur and Pelvic Girdle

5

AP Unilateral Hip

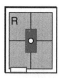

Warning: For possible fractured hip, take AP bilateral hips (preceding page) for comparison purposes.

- 24 × 30 cm L.W. (10 × 12″)
- Grid

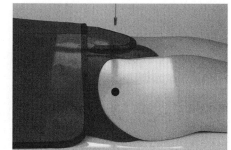

Fig. 5-11 AP hip—CR to femoral neck.

Position
- Supine, leg extended and rotated internally 15°-20° (nontrauma)
- Center femoral neck to CR. Support may be placed under knees for patient comfort.
- Center IR to CR. **Shield gonads** (males and females).

Central Ray: CR ⊥, to femoral neck. (Center slightly lower as needed to include all of orthopedic appliance if present.)

SID: 40-44″ (102-113 cm)

Collimation: Four sides to area of interest

Respiration: Suspend during exposure.

| kV Range: | Analog: 80 ± 5 kV | | | Digital Systems: 80-85 kV | | |

	cm	kV	mA	Time	mAs	SID	Exposure Indicator
S							
M							
L							

Femur and Pelvic Girdle

5

AP Unilateral Hip

Evaluation Criteria
Anatomy Demonstrated:
- Proximal $1/3$ of femur and adjacent parts of pelvic girdle
- Orthopedic appliance in entirety

Position:
- Greater trochanter, femoral head and neck in profile
- Lesser trochanter not visible or minimally only

Exposure:
- Optimal density and contrast
- Sharp trabecular markings clearly demonstrated; no motion

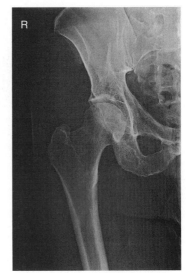

Fig. 5-12 AP hip.

Competency Check: _____

Technologist   Date

Femur and Pelvic Girdle

Lateral Hip (Nontrauma)
(Unilateral "Frog-Leg")

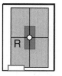

Warning: Do **not** attempt with possible fracture of hip area.

- 24 × 30 cm C.W. (10 × 12″)
- Grid

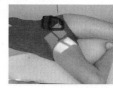

Fig. 5-13 Right hip "frog-leg" lateral (for femoral neck).

Position
- Patient supine
- For femoral neck, flex affected knee and hip, and abduct femur 45° from vertical (places femoral neck near parallel to IR).
- For femoral head, acetabulum, and proximal femoral shaft, oblique patient 35°-45° toward affected side and abduct leg to tabletop if possible. Center hip and neck area to CR.
- Center IR to CR. **Shield gonads** (male and female).

Fig. 5-14 For femoral head and acetabulum and proximal femoral shaft.

Central Ray: CR ⊥, to midfemoral neck or head
SID: 40-44″ (102-113 cm)
Collimation: To proximal femur and hip
Respiration: Suspend during exposure.

kV Range:	Analog: **80 ± 5 kV**	Digital Systems: **80-85 kV**

	cm	kV	mA	Time	mAs	SID	Exposure Indicator
S							
M							
L							

5

Femur and Pelvic Girdle

Lateral Hips (Nontrauma)
(Bilateral "Frog-Leg")

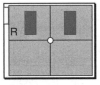

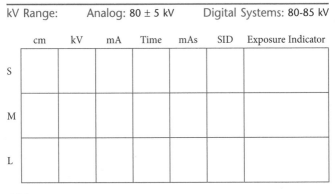

Warning: Do **not** attempt with possible fracture of hip areas.

- 35 × 43 cm C.W. (14 × 17″)
- Grid

Fig. 5-15 Bilateral "frog-leg" (for comparison).

Position

- Supine, centered to CR and IR, flex hips and knees and **abduct both thighs equally** to 45° from vertical* if possible, with feet together
- Ensure **no rotation** of pelvis (ASISs equal distance from table)
- Center IR to CR, **shield gonads** (male and female).

Central Ray: CR ⊥, to level of femoral heads (≈7-8 cm or 3″ inferior to level of ASISs)

SID: 40-44″ (102-113 cm)

Collimation: To IR borders

Respiration: Suspend during exposure.

| kV Range: | Analog: 80 ± 5 kV | | | Digital Systems: 80-85 kV | | |

	cm	kV	mA	Time	mAs	SID	Exposure Indicator
S							
M							
L							

Bontrager Textbook, 8th ed, p. 278.

Femur and Pelvic Girdle

5

AP Bilateral "Frog-Leg"

Evaluation Criteria

Anatomy Demonstrated:

- Femoral heads and necks, acetabulum, and trochanteric anatomy

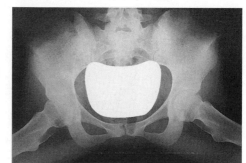

Fig. 5-16 AP bilateral "frog-leg."

Position:

- No rotation evident by symmetry of pelvic bones
- Lesser trochanters equal in size
- Greater trochanters superimposed over femoral necks

Exposure:

- Optimal density and contrast
- Sharp trabecular markings clearly demonstrated; no motion

5

Femur and Pelvic Girdle

Lateral Hip (Trauma Method)

(Axiolateral Inferosuperior Projection [Danelius-Miller Method])

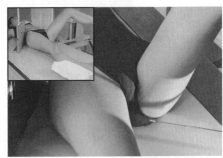

Fig. 5-17 Axiolateral trauma hip (pad under foot).

- 24 × 30 cm C.W. (IR parallel to femur) (10 × 12″)
- Portable grid

Position
- Supine, no rotation of pelvis
- Flex unaffected knee and hip and provide support such as the x-ray tube (use pad or towels for possible **hot collimator**).
- Rotate affected leg internally 15° **unless possible hip fracture.**
- Place vertical grid IR against side just superior to iliac crest with plane of IR perpendicular to CR.

Central Ray: CR horizontal, perpendicular to femoral neck area and IR

SID: 40-44″ (102-113 cm)

Collimation: On four sides to proximal femur area

Respiration: Suspend during exposure.

kV Range:		Analog: 80 ± 5 kV			Digital Systems: 80-85 kV		
	cm	kV	mA	Time	mAs	SID	Exposure Indicator
S							
M							
L							

Bontrager Textbook, 8th ed, p. 284.

Axiolateral Inferosuperior Hip
(Danelius-Miller Method)

Evaluation Criteria

Anatomy Demonstrated:

- Entire femoral head and neck, trochanters, and acetabulum
- Orthopedic appliance in entirety

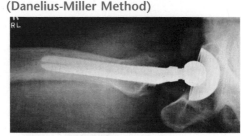

Fig. 5-18 Axiolateral hip.

Competency Check: _____

Technologist   Date

Position:

- Femoral head, neck, and acetabulum demonstrated with little superimposition of opposite hip
- No excessive grid lines present on radiograph.
- Minimal distortion of femoral neck

Exposure:

- Optimal density and contrast
- Use of compensation filter recommended.
- Sharp trabecular markings clearly seen; no motion

AP Pelvis

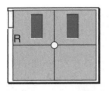

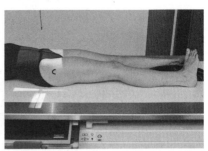

To include proximal femora, pelvic girdle, sacrum, and coccyx

Warning: Do not attempt to rotate legs if fractures involving hips are suspected.

Fig. 5-19 AP pelvis (entire pelvis centered to IR).

Note: For bilateral hips centering, see p. 291.

- 35 × 43 cm C.W. (14 × 17″)
- Grid

Position

- Supine, pelvis centered to centerline, legs extended
- Both feet, knees, and legs equally rotated internally 15° (secure with tape if necessary). Support under knees for comfort.
- Ensure no rotation of pelvis (ASISs equal distance from TT).
- Center IR to CR. (Include entire pelvis.) **Shield gonads** (if it doesn't compromise study).

Central Ray: CR ⊥, midway between ASISs and symphysis pubis (which is about 5 cm or 2″ distal to level of ASISs)

SID: 40-44″ (102-113 cm)

Collimation: On four sides to include entire pelvis

Respiration: Suspend during exposure.

kV Range:	Analog: 80 ± 5 kV			Digital Systems: 80-85 kV		

	cm	kV	mA	Time	mAs	SID	Exposure Indicator
S							
M							
L							

Bontrager Textbook, 8th ed, p. 277.

Femur and Pelvic Girdle

AP Pelvis

Evaluation Criteria

Anatomy Demonstrated:

- Pelvic girdle, L5, sacrum, coccyx, and proximal femora
- Orthopedic appliance in entirety (if present)

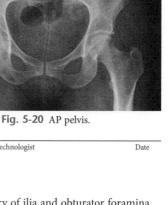

Fig. 5-20 AP pelvis.

Competency Check: _____
Technologist   Date

Position:

- Lesser trochanters generally not visible (nontrauma)
- **No rotation** evident by symmetry of ilia and obturator foramina.

Exposure:

- Optimal density and contrast
- Soft tissue and sharp trabecular markings clearly demonstrated; no motion

5

Femur and Pelvic Girdle

AP Axial Pelvis
("Inlet" and "Outlet" Projections)

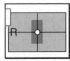

- 35 × 43 cm C.W. (14 × 17")
- Grid

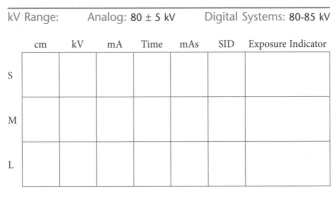

Fig. 5-21 AP axial pelvis.

Fig. 5-22 CR 40° caudal for **inlet.**

Fig. 5-23 CR **cephalad 20° to 35° for males** and **30° to 45° for females—outlet.**

Position
- Supine, patient centered to centerline
- No rotation of pelvis (ASISs the same distance from tabletop)
- Center IR to projected CR. Gonadal shielding may not be possible without obscuring essential anatomy.

Central Ray:
- **Inlet**—CR 40° caudal to level of ASISs, male and female
- **Outlet**—CR: male, 20°-35° cephalad; female, 30°-45° cephalad centered 1-2" (3-5 cm) inferior to symphysis pubis or greater trochanter

SID: 40-44" (102-113 cm)
Collimation: Four sides to area of interest
Respiration: Suspend during exposure.

kV Range:	Analog: 80 ± 5 kV			Digital Systems: 80-85 kV		
	cm	kV	mA	Time	mAs	SID	Exposure Indicator
S							
M							
L							

Bontrager Textbook, 8th ed, pp. 279 and 280.

AP Axial Pelvis
("Inlet" and "Outlet" Projections)

Evaluation Criteria
Anatomy Demonstrated:

- **Inlet:** Pelvic ring or inlet in its entirety
- **Outlet:** Superior/inferior rami of pubes and ramus of ischium

Position:

- **Inlet:** Ischial spines are demonstrated and equal in size; no rotation
- **Outlet:** Obturator foramina are equal in size

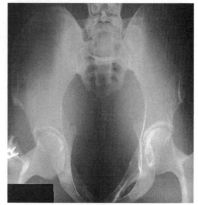

Fig. 5-24 AP axial inlet projection.

Competency Check: _____
                    Technologist   Date

Exposure:

- Optimal density and contrast; no motion
- Pelvic ring is not overexposed

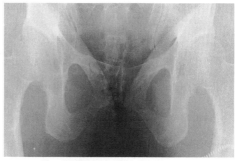

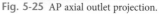

Fig. 5-25 AP axial outlet projection.

Competency Check: _____
                    Technologist   Date

Acetabulum—Posterior Oblique Pelvis
(Judet Method)

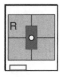

Note: Both sides generally are taken for comparison, either both for upside or both for downside.

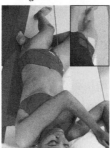

Fig. 5-26 Downside acetabulum.

Fig. 5-27 Upside acetabulum.

- 24 × 30 cm L.W. (10 × 12″) or 35 × 43 cm C.W. (14 × 17″) if both hips must be seen on each projection.
- Grid

Position

- Patient in 45° posterior oblique position, centered for either upside or downside hip joint (dependent on anatomy of interest)
- Place 45° support under elevated side, position arms and legs as shown to maintain this position.

Central Ray:
- **Downside**—CR ⊥, to 2″ (5 cm) distal and 2″ (5 cm) medial to downside ASIS
- **Upside**—CR ⊥ to 2″ (5 cm) distal to upside ASIS

SID: 40-44″ (102-113 cm)

Collimation: Four sides to area of interest

Respiration: Suspend during exposure.

kV Range:	Analog: 80 ± 5 kV	Digital Systems: 80-85 kV

	cm	kV	mA	Time	mAs	SID	Exposure Indicator
S							
M							
L							

Bontrager Textbook, 8th ed, p. 281.

5

Femur and Pelvic Girdle

Acetabulum
(Posterior Oblique [Judet Method])

Evaluation Criteria

Anatomy Demonstrated:

- **Downside:** Anterior rim of acetabulum and posterior ilioischial column
- **Upside:** Posterior rim of acetabulum and anterior iliopubic column

Position:

- **Downside:** Iliac wing elongated and obturator foramina narrowed
- **Upside:** Iliac wing foreshortened and obturator foramina open

Exposure:

- Optimal density and contrast
- Bony margins and trabecular markings are sharp; no motion

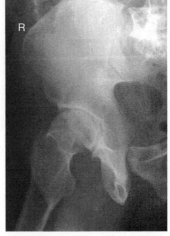

Fig. 5-28 RPO downside visualized.

Competency Check: _____
Technologist   Date

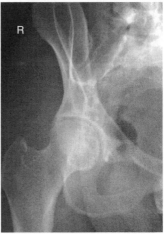

Fig. 5-29 LPO upside visualized.

Competency Check: _____
Technologist   Date

Acetabulum
(PA Axial Oblique Projection [Teufel Method])

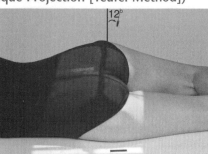

Both sides generally are taken for comparison.
- 24 × 30 cm (10 × 12"), L.W.
- Grid

Fig. 5-30 PA axial oblique.

Position
- Patient semiprone; affected side down
- Rotate body 35°-40° anterior oblique

Central Ray:
- CR 12° cephalad
- 1" (2.5 cm) superior to level of greater trochanter. Approximately 2" (5 cm) lateral to the midsagittal plane.

SID: 40-44" (102-113 cm)

Collimation: Region of acetabulum and proximal femur

kV Range:		Analog: **70-80 kV**			Digital Systems: **80-85 kV**	
	cm	kV	mA	Time	mAs	SID	Exposure Indicator
S							
M							
L							

Bontrager Textbook, 8th ed, p. 282.

Acetabulum
(PA Axial Oblique Projection [Teufel Method])

Evaluation Criteria

Anatomy Demonstrated:

- Superoposterior wall of the acetabulum

Position:

- Fovea capitis with the femoral head in profile
- Obturator foramen open

Exposure:

- Optimal density and contrast; no motion
- Sharp trabecular markings clearly seen

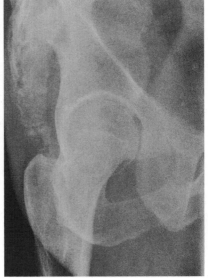

Fig. 5-31 PA axial oblique.

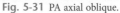

Competency Check: _____

Technologist   Date

Femur and Pelvic Girdle

Pediatric AP and Lateral Hips

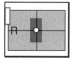

Warning: Do not attempt "frog-leg" lat. with possible hip pathology unless so indicated by a physician after review of AP pelvis radiograph.

- Size determined by patient size; IR C.W.
- Grid >10 cm

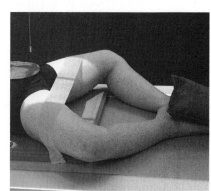

Fig. 5-32 "Frog-leg" lateral hips.

Position (AP and Lateral)

- Supine, pelvis centered to CR and to IR; use **gonadal shields on both male and female.** (Use ovarian shield of appropriate size for female, ensuring that it does not cover hip areas.)
- Immobilize arms and upper body with sandbags, tape, or compression band as needed.

AP: Extend legs and internally rotate 15°.

Frog-Leg Lateral: Flex knees and hips, place feet together and abduct both legs, secure with tape and sandbags.

Central Ray: CR ⊥, centered to level of hips

SID: 40-44″ (102-113 cm)

Collimation: To pelvic margins

Respiration: Full inspiration if crying

kV Range:	Analog: **60-65 kV**	Digital Systems: **65-75 kV**

	cm	kV	mA	Time	mAs	SID	Exposure Indicator
S							
M							
L							

Bontrager Textbook, 8th ed., p. 639.

Chapter 6

Vertebral Column

6

Vertebral Column

(R) Routine, (S) Special

6

Vertebral Column

Intervertebral Foramina and Zygapophyseal Joints

Certain lateral and oblique projections best demonstrate these important foramina and joints of the spine as follows:

	Zygapophyseal Joints	Intervertebral Foramina
Cervical spine	Lateral position	45° anterior oblique (side closest to IR)
Thoracic spine	70° anterior oblique (side closest to IR)	Lateral position
Lumbar spine	45° posterior oblique (side closest to IR)	Lateral position

Topographic Landmarks

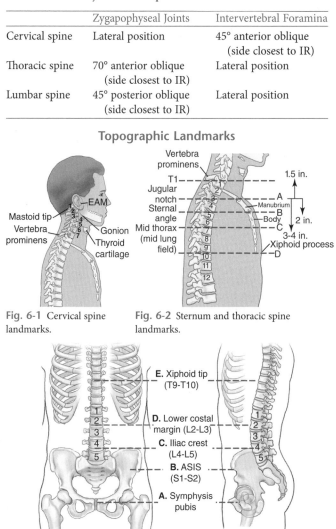

Fig. 6-1 Cervical spine landmarks.

Fig. 6-2 Sternum and thoracic spine landmarks.

Fig. 6-3 Lower spine landmarks.

AP for C1-C2
(Atlas and Axis)

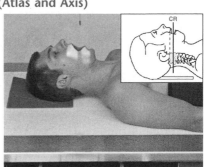

Fig. 6-4 AP open mouth for C1-C2.

- 18 × 24 cm L.W. (8 × 10″)
- Grid
- AEC not recommended because of small field

Position

- Supine, patient centered to CR and centerline
- Adjust head without opening mouth—biting surface of upper incisors (junction of lips) aligned with base of skull (mastoid tips).
- Center IR to CR
- As a last step before making exposure—open mouth wide without moving head (make final check for head alignment).

Central Ray: CR ⊥ through midportion of open mouth (to C1-C2)
SID: 40-44″ (102-113 cm)
Collimation: Close collimation to C1-C2 region
Respiration: Suspend during exposure.

kV Range:	Analog: 70-80 kV				Digital Systems: 75-85 kV	
	cm	kV	mA	Time	mAs	SID	Exposure Indicator
S							
M							
L							

Bontrager Textbook, 8th ed., p. 308.

AP for Dens (Odontoid Process)
(AP Fuchs Method [and PA Judd Method])

R

Warning: Do not attempt on possible cervical trauma.
- 18 × 24 cm L.W. (8 × 10")
- Grid
- AEC not recommended

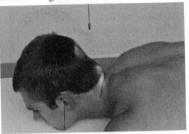

Fig. 6-5 AP Fuchs for dens (within foramen magnum outline).

Position
- Supine or erect, MSP aligned to centerline, no rotation
- Elevate chin until MML is near ⊥ to IR (may require some cephalic CR angle if chin cannot be elevated sufficiently)

Note: May also be taken PA (Judd method) with chin against tabletop, with same CR alignment.

Fig. 6-6 PA Judd method.

- Center IR to exiting CR.

Central Ray: CR parallel to MML directed to tip of mandible (AP)

SID: 40-44" (102-113 cm)

Collimation: Close collimation to C1-C2 region

Respiration: Suspend during exposure.

6

Vertebral Column

kV Range:	Analog: 70-80 kV	Digital Systems: 75-85 kV

	cm	kV	mA	Time	mAs	SID	Exposure Indicator
S							
M							
L							

Oblique Projections, Cervical Spine

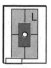

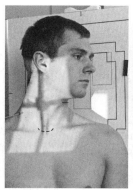

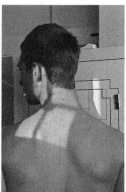

Right and left obliques taken for comparison (as either posterior or anterior obli's); **anterior obli's result in less thyroid dose.**

Fig. 6-11 LPO; CR 15° cephalad.

Fig. 6-12 RAO; CR 15° caudad.

- 18 × 24 cm (8 × 10″) or 24 × 30 cm (10 × 12″), L.W.
- Grid (screen optional for small patient or pediatrics)

Position

- Erect preferred (sitting or standing), entire torso and head turned 45° to IR, C spine aligned to CR (and centerline of IR)
- Raise chin slightly, looking straight ahead (or turn head slightly toward IR to prevent superimposing C1 by mandible).
- Center IR to projected CR.

Central Ray (Posterior Obliques): CR 15°-20° **cephalad,** to enter at C4. **Caudal** angle required for anterior obliques.

SID: 60-72″ (153-183 cm)

Collimation: To C spine region

Respiration: Suspend during exposure.

| kV Range: | Analog: 70-80 kV | | | | Digital Systems: 75-85 kV | |

	cm	kV	mA	Time	mAs	SID	Exposure Indicator
S							
M							
L							

Bontrager Textbook, 8th ed, p. 310.

AP Axial and Oblique Cervical Spine

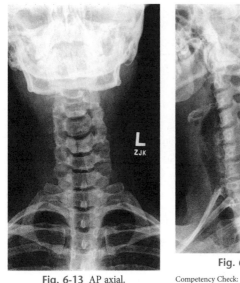

Fig. 6-13 AP axial.

Competency Check: _____
                        Technologist   Date

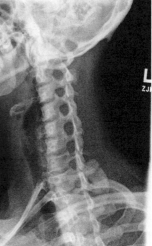

Fig. 6-14 RPO.

Competency Check: _____
                        Technologist   Date

Evaluation Criteria

Anatomy Demonstrated:

- **AP axial:** C3 to T2 vertebral bodies and intervertebral joints
- **Oblique:** Intervertebral foramina open and pedicles
- **LPO/RPO projections:** Demonstrate upside intervertebral foramina
- **LAO/RAO projections:** Demonstrate downside intervertebral foramina

Position:

- **AP axial:** Intervertebral joints open and spinous processes equidistant to midline
- **Oblique: 45° (AP or PA):** Intervertebral foramina uniformly open and pedicles in profile

Exposure:

- Optimal density (brightness) and contrast; no motion
- Soft tissue and bony margins and trabecular markings sharp

6

Vertebral Column

179

Lateral Cervical Spine

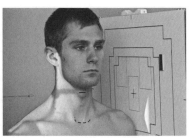

Fig. 6-15 Erect lateral, 183 cm (72″) SID.

- 24 × 30 cm L.W. (10 × 12″)
- Grid (screen optional for small patient or pediatrics)

Position

- Erect (sitting or standing) in lateral position, C spine aligned and centered to CR (and centerline of IR)
- Top of IR ≈1-2″ (3-5 cm) above level of EAM
- Raise chin slightly (to remove mandible angles from spine).
- Relax and depress both shoulders evenly (weights in each hand may be necessary to visualize C7).

Note: See following page for swimmer's lateral if C7 is still not visualized.

Central Ray: CR ⊥, to level of C4 (upper thyroid cartilage)

SID: 60-72″ (153-183 cm) (Longer SID provides for better visualization of C7 because of less divergent rays.)

Collimation: On four sides to C spine region

Respiration: Expose on complete expiration.

	kV Range:	Analog: **70-80 kV**		Digital Systems: **75-85 kV**		

	cm	kV	mA	Time	mAs	SID	Exposure Indicator
S							
M							
L							

Bontrager Textbook, 8th ed, p. 311.

6

Vertebral Column

Lateral Cervicothoracic Spine
Swimmer's (Twining Method) C5-T3 Region

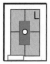

- 24 × 30 cm L.W. (10 × 12″)
- Grid

Position

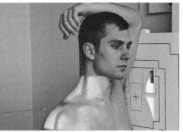

Fig. 6-16 Cervicothoracic (swimmer's) lateral.

- Erect preferred, align C-spine to CR (and centerline of IR).
- Elevate arm and shoulder closest to IR and rotate this shoulder slightly anteriorly or posteriorly.
- Opposite arm down, relax and depress shoulder, with slight opposite rotation (from other shoulder) to separate humeral heads from vertebra. May also be taken in lateral recumbent position with one arm and shoulder down and one up—**Pawlow method.**

Central Ray: CR ⊥, centered to T1 (approximately 1″ [2.5 cm] above level of jugular notch). **Optional** 3°-5° caudad to separate the two shoulders

SID: 60-72″ (153-183 cm)

Collimation: Collimate closely to area of interest

Respiration: Expose on full expiration or orthostatic (breathing) technique.

	cm	kV	mA	Time	mAs	SID	Exposure Indicator
S							
M							
L							

kV Range: Analog: 75-85 kV Digital Systems: 80-95 kV

6

Vertebral Column

Erect Lateral and Cervicothoracic (Swimmer's) Lateral

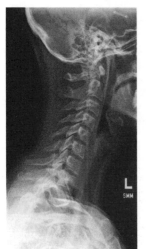

Fig. 6-17 Erect lateral.

Competency Check: _____
                    Technologist   Date

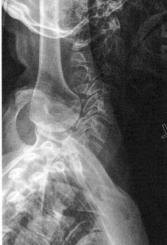

Fig. 6-18 Cervicothoracic (swimmer's) lateral.

Competency Check: _____
                    Technologist   Date

Evaluation Criteria

Anatomy Demonstrated:
- **Lateral:** C1-C7 (minimum) demonstrated
- **Swimmer's:** Vertebral bodies from C5-T3 (minimum) demonstrated

Position:
- **Lateral:** Near superimposition of zygapophyseal joints; no superimposition of mandible on C spine
- **Swimmer's:** Separation of humeral heads from C spine; vertebral bodies in lateral perspective

Exposure:
- Optimal density (brightness) and contrast of lower cervical and upper thoracic spine; no motion
- Soft tissue and bony anatomy visible

Lateral Cervical Spine
Hyperflexion—Hyperextension

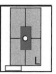

Warning: Do **NOT** attempt on possible trauma patients.
- 24 × 30 cm L.W. (10 × 12″)
- Grid or nongrid

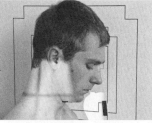

Fig. 6-19 Hyperflexion.

Position
- Erect preferred (sitting or standing) in lateral position, C spine aligned to CR (and centerline of IR)
- Relax and depress shoulders as much as possible.

First IR: Depress chin to touch chest if possible.

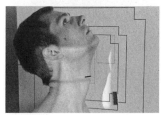

Fig. 6-20 Hyperextension.

Second IR: Elevate chin as far as is comfortable (ensure that entire C spine is included on both projections).

Central Ray: CR ⊥, to C4 (level of upper border of thyroid cartilage)

SID: 60-72″ (153-183 cm)

Collimation: To C spine area

Respiration: Expose on total expiration.

kV Range:	Analog: 70-80 kV			Digital Systems: 75-85 kV		
	cm	kV	mA	Time	mAs	SID	Exposure Indicator
S							
M							
L							

Vertebral Column

6

Hyperflexion and Hyperextension Laterals

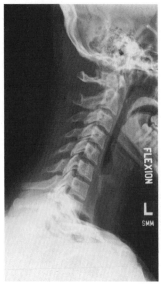

Fig. 6-21 Hyperflexion lateral.

Competency Check: _____
                   Technologist   Date

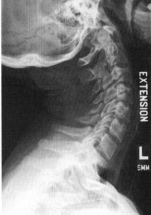

Fig. 6-22 Hyperextension lateral.

Competency Check: _____
                   Technologist   Date

Evaluation Criteria

Anatomy Demonstrated:

- **C1-C7:** Range of motion and ligament stability demonstrated

Position:

- **Hyperflexion:** Spinous processes well separated
- **Hyperextension:** Spinous processes in close proximity

Exposure:

- Optimal density (brightness) and contrast; no motion
- Soft tissue visible and trabecular markings sharp

Vertebral Column

6

184

Cervical Spine—Trauma Series

Warning: Do not remove cervical collar unless so indicated by the physician after viewing horizontal beam lateral.

Horizontal Beam Lateral
- 24 × 30 cm L.W. (10 × 12")
- Grid or nongrid
- SID: 60-72" (153-183 cm)
- CR ⊥, to C4 (upper thyroid cartilage) (top of IR ≈3-5 cm or 1-2" above EAM)

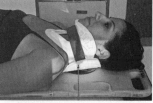
Fig. 6-23 Horizontal beam lateral.

AP
- Depress shoulders.
- 24 × 30 cm L.W. (10 × 12")
- Grid
- **SID:** 40-48" (102-123 cm)
- **CR:** 15°-20° cephalad, to enter at C4

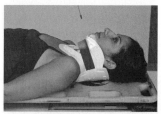
Fig. 6-24 AP axial.

AP Axial Oblique
- 24 × 30 cm (10 × 12") L.W.
- Grid
- **SID:** 40-48" (102-123 cm)
- **CR:** 45° medially (and 15° cephalad if nongrid)
- CR to enter at level of C4

Cervicothoracic Lateral
(Optional projection if needed to visualize C7)
- 24 × 30 cm (10 × 12") L.W.
- Grid
- Elevate shoulder and arm nearest IR. Depress opposite shoulder.
- **SID:** 40-48" (102-123 cm)
- **CR:** IR centered to T1 (approximately 1.5" [2.5 cm] above level of jugular notch)

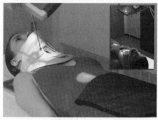
Fig. 6-25 Oblique (both R and L obliques).

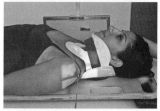
Fig. 6-26 Swimmer's lateral.

6

Vertebral Column

AP Thoracic Spine

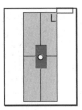

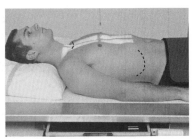

Fig. 6-27 AP thoracic spine.

- 35 × 43 cm L.W. (14 × 17")
- Grid
- Feet at cathode end (anode heel effect)
- Wedge compensation filter recommended to produce uniform density of spine

Position

- Supine, spine aligned and centered to centerline, flex hips and knees to reduce lordotic curvature
- Top of IR 1.5" (3 cm) above shoulder
- Ensure no rotation of thorax or pelvis. Shield radiosensitive tissues.

Central Ray: CR ⊥, to center of IR (at level of T7 as for an AP chest, 3-4" or 8-10 cm below jugular notch)

SID: 40-44" (102-113 cm)

Collimation: Long narrow collimation field to T spine region

Respiration: Expose on expiration for more uniform density.

	cm	kV	mA	Time	mAs	SID	Exposure Indicator
S							
M							
L							

kV Range: Analog: 75-85 kV   Digital Systems: 85-95 kV

Bontrager Textbook, 8th ed, p. 318.

Lateral Thoracic Spine

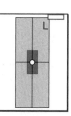

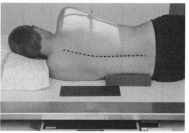

Fig. 6-28 Lateral thoracic spine.

- 35 × 43 cm L.W. (14 × 17")
- Grid
- Lead blocker posterior to patient

Position

- Recumbent, support under head, lateral with hips and knees flexed, arms raised and elbows flexed. Shield radiosensitive tissues.
- Align and center midaxillary plane to centerline
- Top of IR 1.5" (3 cm) above shoulders; no rotation
- Supports should be placed under lower back as needed to straighten and align spine near parallel to tabletop. (A slight natural curvature corresponding to divergent rays is helpful.)

Central Ray: CR ⊥ to thoracic spine, to center of IR (T7)

SID: 40-44" (102-113 cm)

Collimation: Long, narrow collimation field to T spine region

Respiration: Orthostatic (breathing) technique recommended; or expose on expiration

	cm	kV	mA	Time	mAs	SID	Exposure Indicator
S							
M							
L							

kV Range: Analog: 80-90 kV   Digital Systems: 85-95 kV

AP and Lateral Thoracic Spine

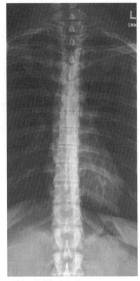

Fig. 6-29 AP thoracic spine.

Competency Check: _____
                      Technologist   Date

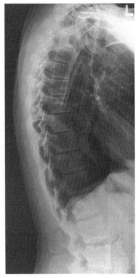

Fig. 6-30 Lateral thoracic spine.

Competency Check: _____
                      Technologist   Date

Evaluation Criteria

Anatomy Demonstrated:

- **AP and lateral:** 12 thoracic bodies, intervertebral joint spaces, and intervertebral foramina

Position:

- **AP:** SC joints equidistant from midline, no rotation
- **Lateral:** Intervertebral joint spaces and intervertebral foramina open

Exposure:

- Optimal density (brightness) and contrast; no motion on AP projection. Breathing technique for lateral projection is desirable.
- Soft tissue visible and trabecular markings sharp

6

Vertebral Column

188

Oblique Thoracic Spine

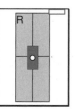

Both oblique projections generally taken for comparison. May also take as anterior obliques (lower breast dose).

- 35 × 43 cm L.W. (14 × 17″)
- Grid

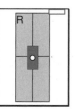

Fig. 6-31 70° RPO (20° from lateral).

Position

- Recumbent, rotated posteriorly 20° from lateral
- Align and center spine to centerline; place arm away from IR behind back and arm closest to IR up in front of head
- Top of IR ≈1 $\frac{1}{2}$″ (3 cm) above shoulders

Central Ray: CR ⊥, to center of IR (T7)

SID: 40-44″ (102-113 cm)

Collimation: Long, narrow collimation field to T spine region

Respiration: Expose on expiration.

	cm	kV	mA	Time	mAs	SID	Exposure Indicator
S							
M							
L							

kV Range: Analog: 75-85 kV   Digital Systems: 85-95 kV

Vertebral Column

6

AP (PA) Lumbar Spine

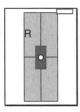

Note: May be taken PA for better opening of intervertebral spaces by divergent rays.

- 30 × 35 cm L.W. (11 × 14″) or 35 × 43 cm (14 × 17″)
- Grid

Position (AP)

- Supine, spine aligned to centerline
- Flex hips and knees (to reduce lordotic curvature).
- No rotation (ASISs same distance from table)
- Center IR to CR.

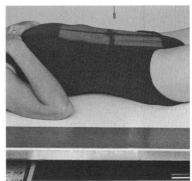

Fig. 6-32 AP lumbar, hips and knees flexed.

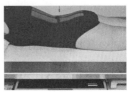

Fig. 6-33 Alternate PA.

Central Ray: CR ⊥, to ≈1″ (2.5 cm) above iliac crest (L3); or center at crest for 35 × 43 cm IR

SID: 40-44″ (102-113 cm)

Collimation: Long, narrow collimation field to L spine region (include SI joints)

Respiration: Expose at end of expiration.

| kV Range: | Analog: 75-85 kV | Digital Systems: 85-95 kV |

	cm	kV	mA	Time	mAs	SID	Exposure Indicator
S							
M							
L							

Bontrager Textbook, 8th ed, p. 335.

AP (PA) Lumbar Spine

Evaluation Criteria
Anatomy Demonstrated:
- T12-S1 (minimum) demonstrated
- Lumbar spine vertebral bodies, intervertebral joints, and transverse processes

Position:
- No rotation evident by symmetry of transverse processes, SI joints, and sacrum.
- Spinous processes are midline.

Exposure:
- Optimal density (brightness) and contrast; no motion
- Soft tissue and sharp trabecular markings clearly demonstrated.

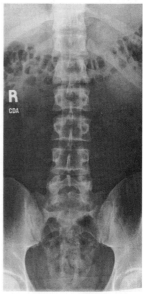

Fig. 6-34 AP lumbar spine.

Competency Check: _____
Technologist   Date

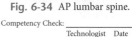

6

Vertebral Column

Lateral Lumbar Spine

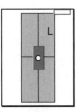

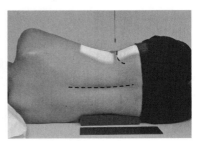

Fig. 6-35 Lateral L spine.

- 30 × 35 or 35 × 43 cm L.W. (11 × 14″ or 14 × 17″)
- Grid
- Feet at cathode end
- Lead blocker, posterior to patient

Position

- Recumbent in true lateral position, flex hips and knees, align and center midaxillary plane to centerline
- Place support under waist as needed to place entire spine parallel to tabletop (see *Note*). Provide support between knees.
- Center IR to CR.

Central Ray: CR ⊥, to spine. CR to level of ≈1″ (2.5 cm) above iliac crest (L3), or at iliac crest for 35 × 43 cm IR

SID: 40-44″ (102-113 cm)

Collimation: Long, narrow collimation field to L spine region

Respiration: Expose at end of expiration.

Note: Patient with wide pelvis and narrow thorax may require a 3°-5° caudal CR angle, even with support under waist. If patient has natural lateral curvature (scoliosis), place "sag" or convexity down.

---

	kV Range:	Analog: **80-90 kV**			Digital Systems: **90-100 kV**	

	cm	kV	mA	Time	mAs	SID	Exposure Indicator
S							
M							
L							

Bontrager Textbook, 8th ed, p. 337.

Vertebral Column

6

Lateral L5-S1, Lumbar Spine

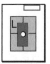

- 18 × 24 cm L.W. (8 × 10″)
- Grid
- Lead blocker posterior to patient

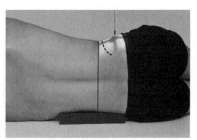

Fig. 6-36 Lateral L5-S1.

Position

- Recumbent in true lateral position, flex hips and knees, midaxillary plane aligned to centerline and CR
- Place support under waist as needed to place entire spine parallel to tabletop. Provide support between knees.
- Center IR to CR.

Central Ray:

- CR ⊥, to IR if entire spine is parallel to table; or 5°-8° caudad if entire spine is not parallel (most often on females). Angle CR to be parallel to the interiliac plane.
- CR to 1.5″ (4 cm) inferior to iliac crest and 2″ (5 cm) posterior to ASIS

SID: 40-44″ (102-113 cm)

Collimation: Collimate closely to area of interest.

Respiration: Suspend during exposure.

6

Vertebral Column

kV Range:	Analog: 85-95 kV			Digital Systems: 90-100 kV		
	cm	kV	mA	Time	mAs	SID	Exposure Indicator
S							
M							
L							

Lateral and Lateral L5-S1 Lumbar Spine

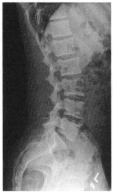

Fig. 6-37 Lateral lumbar spine.

Competency Check: _____
                  Technologist Date

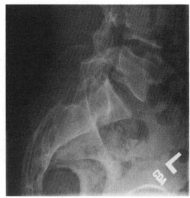

Fig. 6-38 Lateral L5-S1.

Competency Check: _____
                  Technologist   Date

Evaluation Criteria

Anatomy Demonstrated:

- **Lateral:** L1-L4 vertebral bodies, intervertebral joints, and foramina and spinous processes
- **Lateral L5-S1:** Open L4-S1 vertebral bodies, intervertebral joint spaces, and intervertebral foramina

Position:

- **Lateral:** Vertebral column parallel to IR; intervertebral joint spaces and foramina open; no rotation
- **Lateral L5-S1:** Intervertebral joint spaces and intervertebral foramina open; no rotation

Exposure:

- Optimal density (brightness) and contrast; no motion
- Soft tissue visible and bony detail of vertebral bodies, joint spaces, and spinous process

Oblique Lumbar Spine

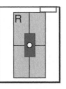

Both oblique projections generally taken for comparison (as either anterior or posterior obliques).

- 11 × 14" L.W. (30 × 35 cm), or 24 × 30 cm (10 × 12")
- Grid

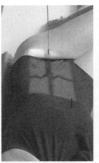

Fig. 6-39 Posterior oblique (45° RPO).

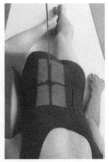

Fig. 6-40 Anterior oblique (45° LAO).

Position

- 45° right and left posterior or anterior obliques (use support angle blocks under pelvis and shoulders to maintain position for posterior obliques)
- Align and center spine to CR and centerline.

Central Ray: CR ⊥, to body of L3 at level of lower costal margin (1-2" or 4-5 cm above iliac crest) and 2" or 5 cm medial to upside ASIS

SID: 40-44" (102-113 cm)

Collimation: To area of interest

Respiration: Suspend during exposure.

Note: 50° oblique is best for L1-L2 zygapophyseal joints, and 30° for L5-S1.

	cm	kV	mA	Time	mAs	SID	Exposure Indicator
S							
M							
L							

kV Range: Analog: 75-85 kV   Digital Systems: 85-95 kV

6

Vertebral Column

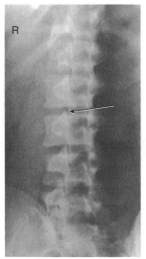

Fig. 6-41 Right posterior oblique.

Competency Check: _____
                    Technologist   Date

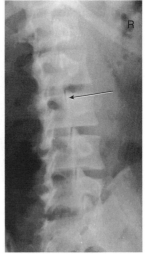

Fig. 6-42 Right anterior oblique.

Competency Check: _____
                    Technologist   Date

Evaluation Criteria

Anatomy Demonstrated:
- **LPO/RPO:** L1-L4 downside zygapophyseal joints. Scottie dog elements visible.
- **LAO/RAO:** L1-L4 upside zygapophyseal joints. Scottie dog elements visible.

Position:
- Zygapophyseal joints and pedicle ("eye") centered on the vertebral body

Exposure:
- Optimal density (brightness) and contrast; no motion
- Soft tissue visible and bony detail of vertebral bodies, joint spaces, and elements of Scottie dog (arrows indicate zygapophyseal joints)

Vertebral Column

6

Scoliosis Series
PA (or AP) Ferguson Method

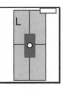

PA greatly reduces breast dose.

- 35 × 43 cm L.W. (14 × 17″) or 35 × 92 cm (14 × 36″)
- Grid
- Compensating filters to produce a more uniform density of spine

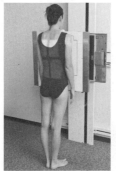

Fig. 6-43 PA without block.

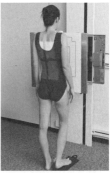

Fig. 6-44 PA with block under foot on convex side of curve.

Position

First IR: Erect, standing or seated, spine aligned and centered to centerline, arms at side, no rotation of pelvis or thorax
- Lower margin of IR 1-2″ (3-5 cm) below iliac crest

Second IR: Place 3- to 4-inch (8- to 10-cm) block under foot (or buttock if seated) on **convex side** of curvature. (Identifies primary deforming curves from compensatory curve.)

Shielding: Use gonad shields and breast shields.

Central Ray: CR ⊥, to center of IR

SID: 40-60″ (102-153 cm); longer SID is recommended

Collimation: Long and narrow to vertebral column region

Respiration: On full expiration

kV Range:	Analog: 80-90 kV	Digital Systems: 85-95 kV

	cm	kV	mA	Time	mAs	SID	Exposure Indicator
S							
M							
L							

6

Vertebral Column

Lumbar Spine
AP (PA) Right and Left Bending

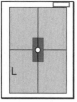

Note: May be taken erect PA to reduce breast dose.

- 35 × 43 cm (14 × 17"), L.W., or 35 × 92 cm (14 × 36")
- Grid
- Compensating filters to produce a more uniform density of spine

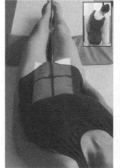

Fig. 6-45 AP, right bending.

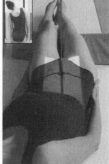

Fig. 6-46 AP, left bending.

Position
- Supine or erect, spine centered to CR and centerline of table
- Bend laterally as far as possible (right then left) without tilting pelvis (pelvis remains stationary and acts as a fulcrum).
- Ensure no rotation of pelvis and upper torso.
- Lower margin of IR 1-2" (3-5 cm) below iliac crest

Central Ray: CR ⊥, to center of IR (higher centering if thoracic spine is area of interest)

SID: 40-60" (102-153 cm)

Collimation: Include vertebral column of interest.

Respiration: Expose at end of expiration.

kV Range:		Analog: 80-90 kV			Digital Systems: 85-95 kV	
	cm	kV	mA	Time	mAs	SID	Exposure Indicator
S							
M							
L							

Bontrager Textbook, 8th ed, p. 343.

6

Vertebral Column

Lumbar Spine
Lateral Hyperflexion and Hyperextension

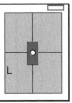

- 35 × 43 cm
  L.W. (14 × 17″)
- Grid
- Lead blocker
  posterior to
  patient

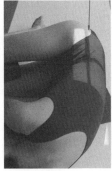

Fig. 6-47 Hyperflexion lateral.

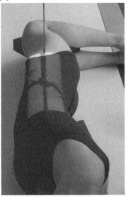

Fig. 6-48 Hyperextension lateral.

Position

- Recumbent or erect, spine centered to table
- Support under waist to align spine parallel to tabletop.
- Hyperflex forward as far as possible, then hyperextend back as far as possible for second IR; maintain true lateral position.
- Lower margin of IR 1-2″ (3-5 cm) below iliac crest

Central Ray: CR ⊥, to center of IR (or to site of fusion if known)
SID: 40-44″ (102-113 cm)
Collimation: On four sides to near borders of IR
Respiration: Expose at end of expiration.

	cm	kV	mA	Time	mAs	SID	Exposure Indicator
S							
M							
L							

kV Range: Analog: 85-95 kV   Digital Systems: 90-100 kV

Vertebral Column

6

Lateral Hyperflexion and Hyperextension

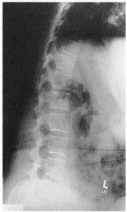

Fig. 6-49 Hyperflexion lateral.

Competency Check: _____
Technologist   Date

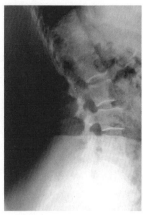

Fig. 6-50 Hyperextension lateral.

Competency Check: _____
Technologist   Date

Evaluation Criteria

Anatomy Demonstrated:
- **Hyperflexion:** Lateral view of lumbar vertebrae in hyperflexion
- **Hyperextension:** Lateral view of lumbar vertebrae in hyperextension

Position:
- **Hyperflexion:** True lateral with no rotation; spaces between spinous processes open
- **Hyperextension:** True lateral with no rotation; spaces between spinous processes closed

Exposure:
- Optimal density (brightness) and contrast; no motion
- Soft tissue visible and bony detail of vertebral bodies, spinous processes, and intervertebral joint spaces

Vertebral Column

AP Axial Sacrum

- 24 × 30 cm L.W.
  (10 × 12″)
- Grid

Fig. 6-51 AP sacrum, CR 15° cephalad.

Position

- Supine, spine centered
  to CR and centerline
- No rotation of pelvis (both ASIS same distance from table)
- Center IR to projected CR. (Shield gonads for males.)

Central Ray: CR 15° cephalad, at 2″ (5 cm) superior to pubic
  symphysis

SID: 40-44″ (102-113 cm)

Collimation: On four sides to area of sacrum

Respiration: Suspend during exposure.

6

Vertebral Column

kV Range:		Analog: 75-80 kV			Digital Systems: 85-90 kV	
	cm	kV	mA	Time	mAs	SID	Exposure Indicator
S							
M							
L							

AP Axial Coccyx

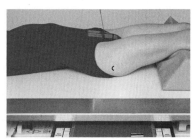

Note: May be done PA with 10° cephalic angle if patient cannot sustain weight on the coccyx area in a supine position.

Urinary bladder should be emptied before procedure is performed.

- 18 × 24 cm L.W. (8 × 10″)
- Grid
- Cautious use of AEC

Fig. 6-52 AP axial coccyx, CR 10° caudad.

Position
- Supine, support under knees, gonad shield for males
- Align and center midsagittal plane to centerline, no rotation
- Center IR to level of projected CR

Central Ray: CR 10° caudad, centered to 2″ (5 cm) superior to symphysis pubis

SID: 40-44″ (102-113 cm)

Collimation: Close collimation to area of coccyx

Respiration: Suspend during exposure.

kV Range:	Analog: 75-80 kV				Digital Systems: 80-85 kV	
	cm	kV	mA	Time	mAs	SID	Exposure Indicator
S							
M							
L							

Bontrager Textbook, 8th ed, p. 346.

AP Axial Sacrum and Coccyx

Evaluation Criteria

Anatomy Demonstrated:

- **AP sacrum:** Nonforeshortened image of sacrum
- **AP coccyx:** Nonforeshortened image of coccyx

Position:

- **AP sacrum:** Sacrum free of superimposition and sacral foramina visible
- **AP coccyx:** Coccyx free of superimposition and not rotated

Exposure:

- Optimal density (brightness) and contrast; no motion
- Soft tissue visible and sharp bony detail

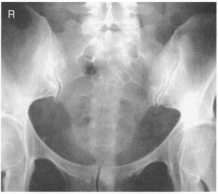

Fig. 6-53 AP sacrum.

Competency Check: _____
Technologist   Date

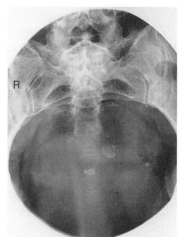

Fig. 6-54 AP coccyx.

Competency Check: _____
Technologist   Date

6

Vertebral Column

203

Lateral Sacrum (and Coccyx)

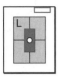

Note: Lateral sacrum and lateral coccyx may be taken as one projection if both sacrum and coccyx are being examined (reduces patient exposure).

- 24 × 30 cm L.W. (10 × 12″)
- Grid
- Lead blocker posterior to patient
- Use of boomerang-type compensating filter is recommended.

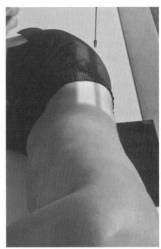

Fig. 6-55 Lateral sacrum.

Position

- Lateral recumbent, hips and knees flexed, true lateral position
- Center sacrum to CR and centerline. (Align patient and IR to correctly centered CR.)

Central Ray (Sacrum): CR ⊥, directed to 3-4″ (8-10 cm) posterior to upside ASIS

SID: 40-44″ (102-113 cm)

Collimation: On four sides to area of sacrum

Respiration: Suspend during exposure.

kV Range:	Analog: 85-95 kV				Digital Systems: 90-100 kV	

	cm	kV	mA	Time	mAs	SID	Exposure Indicator
S							
M							
L							

Bontrager Textbook, 8th ed, p. 347.

6

Vertebral Column

Lateral Coccyx

Note: Lateral sacrum and lateral coccyx are commonly taken as one projection if both sacrum and coccyx are being examined (reduces patient exposure).

- 18 × 24 cm L.W. (8 × 10″)
- Grid
- Lead blocker posterior to patient
- Cautious use of AEC

Position

- Lateral recumbent, with hips and knees flexed 90°, true lateral position

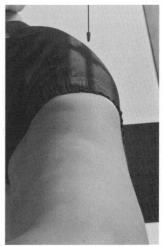

Fig. 6-56 Lateral coccyx.

- Center coccyx to CR and centerline of table (remember the coccyx is located superficially between buttocks slightly superior to level of greater trochanter).
- Center IR to CR.

Central Ray: CR ⊥, to 2″ (5 cm) inferior to level of ASIS and 3-4″ (8-10 cm) posterior

SID: 40-44″ (102-113 cm)

Collimation: To area of distal sacrum and coccyx

Respiration: Suspend during exposure.

	cm	kV	mA	Time	mAs	SID	Exposure Indicator
S							
M							
L							

kV Range: Analog: 75-85 kV   Digital Systems: 85-90 kV

6

Vertebral Column

Lateral Sacrum and Coccyx

Evaluation Criteria

Anatomy Demonstrated:
- Lateral view of sacrum and coccyx
- Lateral view of L5-S1 intervertebral joint

Position:
- No rotation evident by greater sciatic notches and femoral heads superimposed
- Entire sacrum and coccyx included

Exposure:
- Optimal density (brightness) and contrast; no motion
- Soft tissue and sharp trabecular markings clearly demonstrated

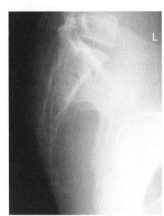

Fig. 6-57 Lateral sacrum and coccyx.

Competency Check: _____
Technologist   Date

Vertebral Column

Sacroiliac Joints
AP Axial

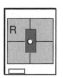

- 24 × 30 cm L.W.
  (10 × 12″)
- Grid

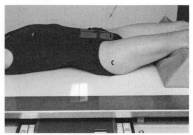

Fig. 6-58 AP axial SI joints (CR 30°-35° cephalad).

Position
- Supine, center patient to centerline
- No rotation of pelvis (ASISs the same distance from tabletop)
- Center IR to projected CR. **Shield gonads** for males.

Central Ray: CR 30° (males) and 35° (females) cephalad, 2″ (5 cm) below level of ASIS

SID: 40-44″ (102-113 cm)

Collimation: Four sides to area of interest

Respiration: Suspend during exposure.

6

Vertebral Column

kV Range:		Analog: 80-90 kV		Digital Systems: 90-100 kV		
	cm	kV	mA	Time	mAs	SID	Exposure Indicator
S							
M							
L							

Sacroiliac Joints
Posterior Oblique Projections (Bilateral)

- 24 × 30 cm L.W. (10 × 12″)
- Grid
- Bilateral for comparison

Position
- Patient in 25°-30° posterior oblique with side of interest elevated (use support to maintain this position)
- Align elevated SI joint to CR and to centerline (1″ [2.5 cm] medial to upside ASIS)
- Center IR to CR.
- **Shield gonads** for males.

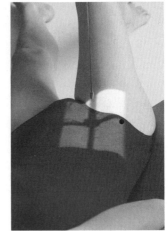

Fig. 6-59 25°-30° LPO for upside (right) joint.

Central Ray: CR ⊥, to 1″ (2.5 cm) medial to elevated ASIS

SID: 40-44″ (102-113 cm)

Collimation: Four sides to area of interest

Respiration: Suspend during exposure.

Note: CR may be angled 15°-20° cephalad to best demonstrate the distal part of joint.

		kV Range:	Analog: 80-90 kV		Digital Systems: 85-95 kV		
	cm	kV	mA	Time	mAs	SID	Exposure Indicator
S							
M							
L							

Bontrager Textbook, 8th ed, p. 350.

Posterior Oblique SI Joint

Evaluation Criteria
Anatomy Demonstrated:
• Open upside SI joint

Position:
• **LPO:** Right SI joint open;
  no overlap of iliac wing
  and sacrum
• **RPO:** Left SI joint open;
  no overlap of iliac wing
  and sacrum

Exposure:
• Optimal density
  (brightness) and contrast;
  no motion
• Soft tissue and sharp
  trabecular markings
  clearly demonstrated

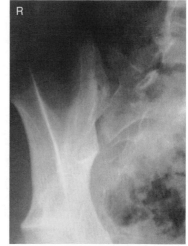

Fig. 6-60 LPO projection of
(right) SI joint.

Competency Check: _____
                    Technologist   Date

Chapter 7

Bony Thorax

(R) Routine, (S) Special

Bony Thorax

7

Bony Thorax—Positioning Considerations

Sternum

The routine for a sternum generally includes a lateral and an oblique wherein the sternum is shifted to the left of the spine and is superimposed over the homogeneous heart shadow. A 15°-20° RAO achieves this best. An orthostatic-breathing technique generally is used to blur out the lung markings and the ribs overlying the sternum. If preferred, exposure can also be made on suspended expiration.

Ribs

Each technologist should determine the preferred routine for his or her department.

Two-Image Routine

One suggested two-image routine is an **AP or PA** with the area of injury closest to the image receptor (IR) (above or below diaphragm) and an **oblique** projection of the axillary ribs on the side of injury. Therefore the oblique for this routine on an injury to the left anterior ribs would be an RAO shifting the spine away from the area of injury and to increase visibility of the left axillary ribs. The oblique for an injury to the right posterior ribs would be an RPO wherein the spine again is rotated away from the area of injury.

Three-Image Routine

Another three-image routine required in some departments for all rib trauma consists of **AP above diaphragm** or **AP below diaphragm** and **RPO** and **LPO** of the site of injury.

Above and Below Diaphragm

The location of the injury site in relationship to the diaphragm is important for all routines. Those injuries above the diaphragm require less exposure (nearer to a chest technique) when taken on **inspiration** and those below the diaphragm require an exposure nearer to that of an abdomen technique when taken on **expiration.**

7

Right Anterior Oblique (RAO) Sternum

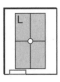

- 24 × 30 cm L.W. (10 × 12″)
- Grid
- Orthostatic-breathing technique or suspended expiration
- AEC not recommended

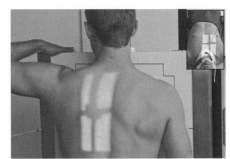

Fig. 7-1 Erect 15°-20° RAO sternum (*insert:* trauma option).

Bony Thorax

7

Position

- Erect (preferred) or semiprone, turned 15°-20° with right side down. (A thin-chested patient requires slightly more obliquity than a thick-chested patient.)
- Center sternum to CR at midline of table or IR holder

Central Ray: CR ⊥, to midsternum (midway between jugular notch and xiphoid process)

SID: 40-44″ (102-113 cm)

Collimation: Long, narrow collimation field to region of sternum

Respiration: Orthostatic-breathing technique of 2-3 seconds or suspend upon expiration

| kV Range: | Analog: 65-75 kV | | | | Digital Systems: 70-80 kV | |

	cm	kV	mA	Time	mAs	SID	Exposure Indicator
S							
M							
L							

Bontrager Textbook, 8th ed., p. 362.

Lateral Sternum

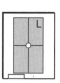

- 24 × 30 cm L.W. (10 × 12″) or 30 × 35 cm (11 × 14″)
- Grid
- AEC not recommended
- Place lead blocker anterior to sternum (for recumbent position)

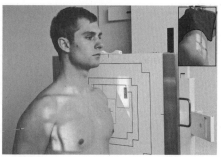

Fig. 7-2 Lateral, erect sternum (trauma option).

Position

- Erect (seated or standing), or recumbent lying on side with vertical CR; or supine with cross-table CR for severe trauma
- Draw shoulders and arms back.
- Align sternum to CR at midline of IR holder.
- Top of IR 1.5″ (4 cm) superior to level of jugular notch

Central Ray: CR ⊥, to midsternum

SID: 60-72″ (153-183 cm)

Collimation: Long, narrow collimation field to region of sternum

Respiration: Expose upon full inspiration.

kV Range:	Analog: 70-75 kV	Digital Systems: 75-80 kV

	cm	kV	mA	Time	mAs	SID	Exposure Indicator
S							
M							
L							

Bony Thorax

7

Oblique (RAO) Sternum

Evaluation Criteria
Anatomy Demonstrated:
- Entire sternum superimposed on heart shadow

Position:
- Correct rotation, sternum visualized alongside vertebral column

Exposure:
- 2- to 3-second exposure using breathing technique; lung markings appear blurred
- Optimal contrast and density (brightness) to visualize entire sternum

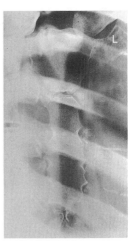

Fig. 7-3 RAO sternum.

Competency Check: _____
Technologist   Date

7

Lateral Sternum

Anatomy Demonstrated:
- Entire sternum

Position:
- No rotation, sternum visualized with no superimposition on the ribs
- Shoulders and arms drawn back

Exposure:
- No motion, sharp bony margins
- Optimal contrast and density (brightness) to visualize entire sternum

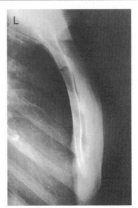

Fig. 7-4 Lateral sternum. (From Frank ED, Long BW, Smith BJ: Merrill's atlas of radiographic positioning and procedures, ed 12, St. Louis, 2012, Elsevier.)

Competency Check: _____
Technologist   Date

Sternoclavicular Joints PA and Anterior Oblique Projections

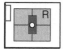

- 18 × 24 cm C.W. (8 × 10″)
- Grid

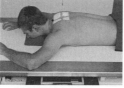

Fig. 7-5 Bilateral PA.

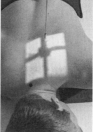

Fig. 7-6 RAO, 10°-15° oblique, CR ⊥ (both obliques commonly taken for comparison).

Position

PA: Prone or erect, midsagittal plane to centerline of CR
- Turn head to side, no rotation of thorax
- Center **IR** to **CR**

Oblique: Rotate thorax 10°-15° to shift vertebrae away from sternum (best visualizes **downside** SC joint). **RAO** will demonstrate the right SC joint. **LAO** will demonstrate the left SC joint.

Less obliquity (5°-10°) will best visualize the upside SC joint next to spine.

Central Ray:
- **PA:** Level of T2-T3. CR ⊥ to MSP and ≈7 cm (3″) distal to vertebra prominens (3 cm or 1.5″ inferior to jugular notch)
- **Oblique:** Level of T2-T3. CR ⊥, to ≈5 cm (2″) lateral to MSP (toward elevated side) and ≈7 cm (3″) distal to vertebra prominens

SID: 40-44″ (102-113 cm)

Collimation: To region of sternoclavicular joints with four-sided collimation

Respiration: Suspend respiration upon expiration.

kV Range:	Analog: 65-70 kV	Digital Systems: 70-75 kV

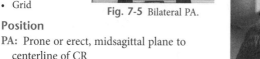

	cm	kV	mA	Time	mAs	SID	Exposure Indicator
S							
M							
L							

Bony Thorax

7

Sternoclavicular (SC) Joints—PA

Evaluation Criteria
Anatomy Demonstrated:
- Lateral aspect of manubrium and medial portion of clavicles visualized lateral to vertebral column

Position:
- No rotation, equal distance of SC joints from vertebral column

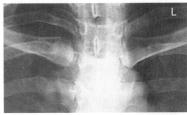

Fig. 7-7 PA SC joints.

Competency Check: _____
                     Technologist   Date

Exposure:
- No motion, sharp bony margins
- SC joints visualized through ribs and lungs
- Optimal contrast and density (brightness) to visualize S.C. joints

---

SC Joints—Anterior Oblique

Anatomy Demonstrated:
- Manubrium and medial clavicles and downside SC joints are visualized

Position:
- Patient rotated 15°, correct rotation best demonstrates downside SC joint with no superimposition of vertebral column

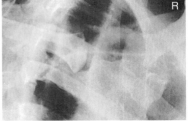

Fig. 7-8 15° RAO.

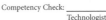

Competency Check: _____
                     Technologist   Date

Exposure:
- No motion, sharp bony margins
- Contrast and density (brightness) sufficient to visualize SC joint through ribs and lungs

Bony Thorax

7

216

AP or PA (Bilateral) Ribs—Above Diaphragm

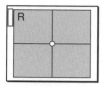

Generally taken as AP for posterior ribs and PA for anterior ribs.

- 35 × 43 cm (14 × 17″) C.W. or L.W. (unilateral study or narrow chest dimensions)
- Grid

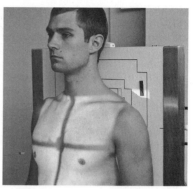

Fig. 7-9 AP bilateral ribs (above diaphragm).

Position

- Erect, or recumbent, midsagittal plane to centerline and CR
- Top of IR ≈1.5″ (4 cm) above shoulders
- Roll shoulders forward, no rotation
- Ensure that thorax is centered to IR (bilateral study).

Central Ray: CR ⊥, to center of IR and 3 or 4″ (8 to 10 cm) below jugular notch (level of T7)

SID: 72″ (183 cm) erect; 40-48″ (102-123 cm) recumbent

Collimation: Collimate to region of interest.

Respiration: Expose on **inspiration** (diaphragm down).

	cm	kV	mA	Time	mAs	SID	Exposure Indicator
S							
M							
L							

kV Range: Analog: 65-75 kV   Digital Systems: 75-85 kV

Bony Thorax

7

AP Ribs (Bilateral)—Below Diaphragm

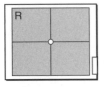

- 35 × 43 cm (14 × 17″) C.W or L.W. (unilateral study or narrow chest dimensions)
- Grid

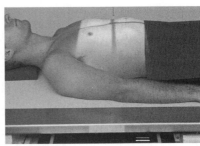

Fig. 7-10 AP bilateral ribs (below diaphragm).

Position
- Erect, or recumbent, MSP to centerline of table and IR (and CR)
- Inferior margin of IR at iliac crest
- Ensure that both lateral margins of thorax are included (bilateral study).
- **Shield gonads** for male and female.

Note: Some routines include only unilateral ribs of affected side.
Central Ray: CR ⊥, centered to IR (level of approximately T9-T10, xiphoid process)
SID: 72″ (183 cm) erect; 40-44″ (102-113 cm) recumbent
Collimation: Collimate to region of interest.
Respiration: Expose on **expiration** (diaphragm up).

| kV Range: | Analog: 70-80 kV | | | Digital Systems: 80-90 kV | | |

	cm	kV	mA	Time	mAs	SID	Exposure Indicator
S							
M							
L							

Bontrager Textbook, 8th ed, pp. 366 and 368.

Ribs—AP or PA

(Above and below diaphragm)

Evaluation Criteria
Anatomy Demonstrated:
Above diaphragm
- Ribs 1-10 visualized

Below diaphragm
- Ribs 9-12 visualized

Position:
- No rotation, lateral rib margins equal distance from vertebral column

Exposure:
- No motion, sharp bony margins
- Contrast and density (brightness) appropriate to visualize ribs 1-10 above diaphragm and 9-12 below diaphragm

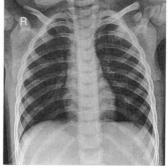

Fig. 7-11 AP above diaphragm.

Competency Check: _____
                    Technologist   Date

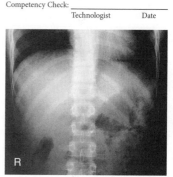

Fig. 7-12 AP below diaphragm.

Competency Check: _____
                    Technologist   Date

Bony Thorax

7

Anterior Oblique Upper Axillary Ribs—RAO

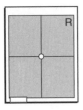

- 35 × 43 cm (14 × 17") or 30 × 35 cm (11 × 14") L.W (see *Note*)
- Grid

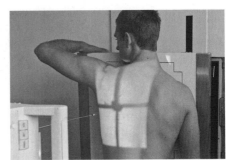

Fig. 7-13 45° RAO above diaphragm—bilateral, right anterior injury (to shift spine away from injury).

Position
- Erect, or recumbent if needed (erect preferred)
- Oblique 45°, rotate spine away from area of interest
- Involved region of thorax is centered to IR with top of IR ≈4 cm (1.5") above shoulders

Note: Some routines indicate unilateral oblique only of affected side with smaller IR placed lengthwise.

Central Ray: CR ⊥, to center of IR (level of T7)

SID: 72" (183 cm) erect, 40-44" (102-113 cm) recumbent

Collimation: Collimate to region of interest.

Respiration: Above diaphragm—expose on **inspiration.**

kV Range:	Analog: 65-75 kV				Digital Systems: 75-85 kV	
	cm	kV	mA	Time	mAs	SID	Exposure Indicator
S							
M							
L							

Bontrager Textbook, 8th ed, pp. 369 and 370.

Posterior Oblique Lower Axillary Ribs—LPO

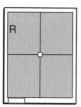

- 35 × 43 cm (14 × 17″) or
  30 × 35 cm (11 × 14″) L.W
- Grid

Position
- Erect or recumbent
  (recumbent preferred)
- Top of IR ≈1.5″ (4 cm) above
  shoulders
- Rotate 45° from AP, arm
  closest to IR up, resting on
  head; opposite hand on waist
  with arm away from body

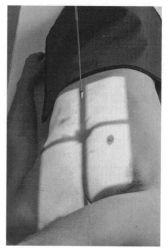

Fig. 7-14 45° LPO (below diaphragm).

Central Ray: CR ⊥, centered to IR (level of T7)
SID: 72″ (183 cm) erect, 40-44″ (102-113 cm) recumbent
Collimation: Collimate to region of interest.
Respiration: Below diaphragm—expose upon **expiration.**

Bony Thorax

7

	cm	kV	mA	Time	mAs	SID	Exposure Indicator
S							
M							
L							

kV Range:	Analog: 70-80 kV	Digital Systems: 80-90 kV

Anterior or Posterior Oblique Axillary Ribs

(Above and below diaphragm)

Evaluation Criteria
Anatomy Demonstrated:
- **LPO/RAO:** Visualizes left axillary ribs
- **RPO/LAO:** Visualizes right axillary ribs
- Ribs 1-10 seen above diaphragm
- Ribs 9-12 seen below diaphragm
- Axillary portion of ribs projected without superimposition

Position:
- 45° oblique should visualize axillary ribs in profile with spine shifted away from area of interest

Exposure:
- No motion, sharp bony margins
- Optimum contrast and density (brightness) visualizes ribs through lungs and heart shadow for above diaphragm, and through dense abdominal organs for below diaphragm

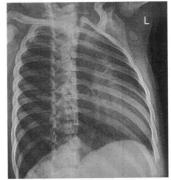

Fig. 7-15 LPO above diaphragm.

Competency Check: _____
Technologist   Date

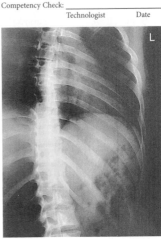

Fig. 7-16 LPO below diaphragm.

Competency Check: _____
Technologist   Date

Chapter 8

Skull, Facial Bones, and Paranasal Sinuses

8

Mandible

Temporomandibular Joints

Paranasal Sinuses

(R) Routine, (S) Special

Cranial landmarks and positioning lines used in skull and facial bones positioning.

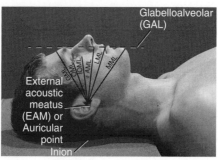

Fig. 8-1 Positioning lines.

A. Glabellomeatal line (**GML**)
B. Orbitomeatal line (**OML**)
C. Infraorbitomeatal line (**IOML**) (Reid's base line, or "base line," base of cranium)
D. Acanthiomeatal line (**AML**)
E. Lips-meatal line (**LML**) (used for modified Waters)
F. Mentomeatal line (**MML**) (used for Waters)

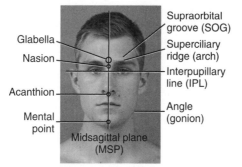

Fig. 8-2 Cranial landmarks.

AP (PA) Axial Skull
AP Towne (or PA Haas Method)

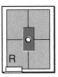

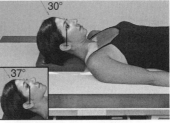

Fig. 8-3 AP axial (Towne)—CR 30° caudad to OML.

- 24 × 30 cm L.W. (10 × 12″)
- Grid

Position
- Seated erect, or supine, midsagittal plane aligned to CR and centerline, perpendicular to IR; no rotation or tilt
- Depress chin to bring OML or IOML perpendicular to IR.
- Center IR to projecting CR.

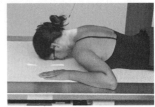

Fig. 8-4 PA axial (Haas method), OML ⊥ CR 25° cephalad, through level of EAMs.

Central Ray:
- CR 30° caudad to OML; or 37° caudad to IOML
- CR to ≈2.5″ or 6 cm above glabella (through 2 cm or 0.75″ superior to level of EAMs)

SID: 40-44″ (102-113 cm)

Collimation: On four sides to skull margins

Respiration: Suspend during exposure.

Note: PA Haas (p. 436 in text) is an alternate to AP Towne. Adjust head to bring OML ⊥ to IR.

8

| kV Range: | Analog: 70-80 kV | | Digital Systems: 80-85 kV | | | |

	cm	kV	mA	Time	mAs	SID	Exposure Indicator
S							
M							
L							

Bontrager Textbook, 8th ed, p. 411.

AP Axial
(Modified Towne Method)

Evaluation Criteria

Anatomy Demonstrated:

- Occipital bone, petrous pyramids, and foramen magnum

Position:

- Dorsum sellae within foramen magnum
- **No rotation** evident by symmetry of petrous pyramids

Exposure:

- Optimal density (brightness) and contrast to visualize occipital bone
- Sharp bony margins; no motion

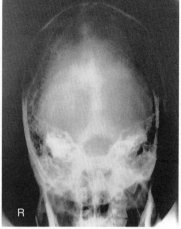

Fig. 8-5 AP axial skull.

Competency Check: _____
                       Technologist   Date

Skull, Facial Bones, and Paranasal Sinuses

8

Lateral Skull

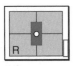

- 24 × 30 cm C.W.
  (10 × 12″)
- Grid

Position
- Seated erect or semiprone on table
- No rotation or tilt, midsagittal plane parallel to IR, and IPL perpendicular to IR
- Adjust chin to place IOML parallel to upper and lower IR edges
- Center IR to CR.

Central Ray: CR ⊥ to IR, ≈2″ (5 cm) superior to EAM
SID: 40-44″ (102-113 cm)
Collimation: On four sides to skull margins
Respiration: Suspend during exposure.

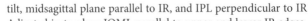

Fig. 8-6 Lateral skull.

kV Range: Analog: 70-80 kV   Digital Systems: 80-85 kV

	cm	kV	mA	Time	mAs	SID	Exposure Indicator
S							
M							
L							

Bontrager Textbook, 8th ed, p. 412.

Skull, Facial Bones, and Paranasal Sinuses

8

Lateral Skull

Evaluation Criteria
Anatomy Demonstrated:
- Superimposed cranial halves
- Entire sella turcica and dorsum sellae

Position:
- **No tilt**, evident by superimposition of orbital plates (roofs)
- **No rotation**, evident by superimposition of greater wings of sphenoid and mandibular rami

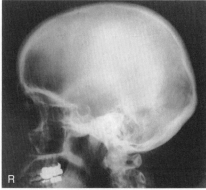

Fig. 8-7 Lateral skull.

Competency Check: _____

                    Technologist   Date

Exposure:
- Optimal density (brightness) and contrast to visualize sellar structures
- Sharp bony margins; no motion

Skull, Facial Bones, and Paranasal Sinuses

8

229

PA (0° and 15°) Caldwell Skull

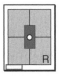

Note: Some departmental routines include a 0° PA to better demonstrate the frontal bone in addition to the 15° PA axial Caldwell.

- 24 × 30 cm L.W. (10 × 12″)
- Grid

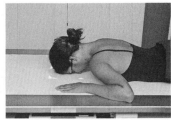

Fig. 8-8 PA—0°.

Position

- Seated erect, or prone on table, head aligned to CR and centerline of IR
- With forehead and nose resting on tabletop, adjust head to place OML perpendicular to IR.

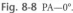
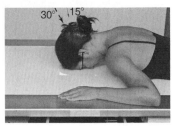

Fig. 8-9 PA axial—15° Caldwell.

- No rotation or tilt, midsagittal plane perpendicular to IR
- Center IR to projected CR.

Central Ray:
- PA 0°: CR ⊥ to IR, centered to exit at glabella
- PA axial (Caldwell): CR 15° caudad to OML, centered to exit at nasion (25°-30° best demonstrates orbital margins)

SID: 40-44″ (102-113 cm)

Collimation: On four sides to skull margins

Respiration: Suspend during exposure.

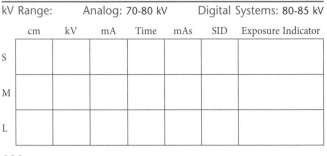

kV Range:		Analog: 70-80 kV		Digital Systems: 80-85 kV		
	cm	kV	mA	Time	mAs	SID	Exposure Indicator
S							
M							
L							

8

PA (0°) and PA Axial Caldwell (15° Caudad)

Evaluation Criteria

Anatomy Demonstrated:
- **PA 0°:** Frontal bone and crista galli demonstrated without distortion
- **PA axial 15°:** Greater/lesser wings of sphenoid, frontal bone, and superior orbital fissures

Position:
- **PA 0°:** Petrous ridges at level of superior orbital margin. No rotation; equal distance between orbits and lateral skull
- **PA axial 15°:** Petrous ridges projected in lower $\frac{1}{3}$ of orbits. No rotation; equal distance between orbits and lateral skull

Exposure:
- Optimal density (brightness) and contrast to visualize frontal bone and surrounding structures
- Sharp bony margins; no motion

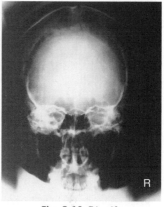

Fig. 8-10 PA—0°.

Competency Check: _____
Technologist   Date

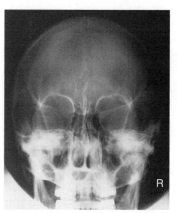

Fig. 8-11 PA axial—15° Caldwell.

Competency Check: _____
Technologist   Date

Skull, Facial Bones, and Paranasal Sinuses

8

231

Submentovertex (SMV) Skull

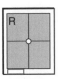

- 24 × 30 cm L.W. (10 × 12″)
- Grid
- AEC optional

Position

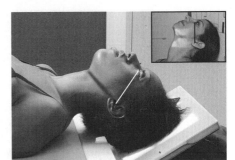

Fig. 8-12 SMV—CR ⊥ to IOML.

- Seated erect or supine with head extended over end of table resting top of head against grid IR (may tilt table up slightly)
- Adjust IR and head to place IOML parallel to IR.
- Ensure no rotation or tilt.
- Center IR to CR.

Central Ray: CR angled to be ⊥ to IOML, centered to 0.75″ (2 cm) anterior to level of EAMs (midpoint between angles of mandible)

Note: If patient cannot extend head this far, adjust CR as needed to remain perpendicular to IOML.

SID: 40-44″ (102-113 cm)

Collimation: On four sides to skull margins

Respiration: Suspend during exposure.

	cm	kV	mA	Time	mAs	SID	Exposure Indicator
S							
M							
L							

kV Range: Analog: 75-85 kV   Digital Systems: 80-90 kV

Submentovertex (SMV) Skull

Evaluation Criteria

Anatomy Demonstrated:

- Base of skull, including mandible and occipital bone
- Foramen ovale and spinosum

Position:

- Mandibular condyles are anterior to the petrous bones
- **No tilt;** equal distance between mandibular condyles and lateral skull
- **No rotation;** MSP parallel to edge of radiograph

Exposure:

- Optimal density and contrast (brightness) to visualize outline of foramen magnum
- Sharp bony margins; no motion

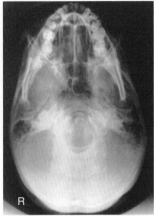

Fig. 8-13 SMV.

Competency Check: _____
                    Technologist   Date

Skull, Facial Bones, and Paranasal Sinuses

8

233

Lateral Trauma Skull

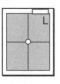

Skull, Facial Bones, and Paranasal Sinuses

Warning: Do **NOT** elevate or move patient's head before cervical spine injuries have been ruled out.
- 24 × 30 cm C.W. (10 × 12″)
- Grid

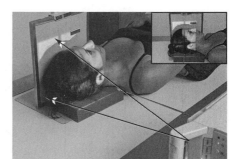

Fig. 8-14 Lateral, with possible spinal injury.

Position

- Supine, without removing cervical collar if present
- With possible spinal injury, move patient to back edge of table and place IR about 1″ (2.5 cm) below tabletop and posterior skull (move floating tabletop forward).
- Center IR to horizontal beam CR (to include entire skull).
- Ensure no rotation or tilt.

Central Ray: CR horizontal, ⊥ to IR, centered to ≈2″ (5 cm) superior to EAM

SID: 40-44″ (102-113 cm)

Collimation: On four sides to skull margins

Respiration: Suspend respiration.

8

| kV Range: | Analog: 70-80 kV | | | Digital Systems: 80-85 kV | | |

	cm	kV	mA	Time	mAs	SID	Exposure Indicator
S							
M							
L							

AP Trauma Skull Series

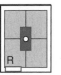

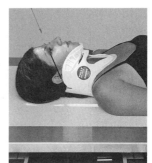

Fig. 8-15 AP—0° to OML.
CR—parallel to OML
—centered to glabella

Warning: With possible spine or severe head injuries, take all projections AP without moving head or without removing cervical collar if present.

- 24 × 30 cm L.W. (10 × 12″)
- Grid (Bucky)

Position

- Patient carefully moved onto x-ray table in supine position
- All projections taken as is without moving head

SID: 40-44″ (102-113 cm)

Collimation: On four sides to skull margins

Respiration: Suspend during exposure, or take "as is."

CR Angle and Centering

- As indicated under each photo
- IR centered to projected CR

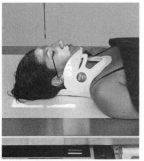

Fig. 8-16 AP reverse Caldwell.
CR—15° cephalad to OML
—centered to nasion

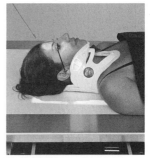

Fig. 8-17 AP axial (Towne).
CR—30° caudad to OML
—centered to midpoint between EAMs

Skull, Facial Bones, and Paranasal Sinuses

8

Evaluation Criteria

Anatomy Demonstrated:

- Superimposed cranial halves
- Entire sella turcica and dorsum sellae

Position:

- No rotation or tilt (see p. 229 for specific criteria)

Exposure:

- Optimal density (brightness) and contrast to visualize sellar structures
- Sharp bony margins; no motion

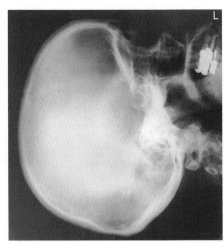

Fig. 8-18 Lateral trauma skull.

Competency Check: _____

Technologist   Date

8

Trauma AP (0°) and AP Axial (15° Cephalad) Projections

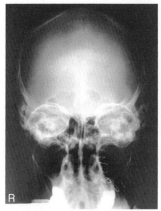

Fig. 8-19 AP—0° to OML.

Competency Check: _____
Technologist   Date

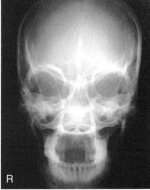

Fig. 8-20 AP axial ("reverse" Caldwell) (15° cephalad).

Competency Check: _____
Technologist   Date

Evaluation Criteria

Anatomy Demonstrated:

- **AP 0°:** Frontal bone and crista galli demonstrated (magnified because of OID)
- **AP axial 15°:** Greater/lesser wings of sphenoid, frontal bone, and superior orbital fissures (magnified)

Position:

- **AP 0°:** Petrous ridges at level of superior orbital margin. **No rotation;** equal distance between orbits and lateral skull
- **AP axial 15°:** Petrous ridges projected in lower $\frac{1}{3}$ of orbits. **No rotation;** equal distance between orbits and lateral skull

Exposure:

- Optimal density (brightness) and contrast to visualize frontal bone and surrounding structures
- Sharp bony margins; no motion

8

Facial Bones—Lateral

- 8 × 10″ L.W.
  (18 × 24 cm)
- Grid

Position
- Seated erect or
  semiprone on
  table
- No rotation or
  tilt, midsagittal
  plane parallel to
  IR, IPL perpendicular to IR

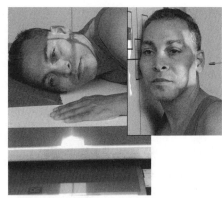

Fig. 8-21 Lateral facial bones.

- Adjust chin to place IOML parallel to top and bottom edge of IR.
- Center IR to CR.

Central Ray: CR ⊥ to IR, centered to midway between EAM and
outer canthus

SID: 40-44″ (102-113 cm)

Collimation: On four sides to area of facial bones

Respiration: Suspend during exposure.

8

kV Range:	Analog: 65-75 kV	Digital Systems: 70-80 kV

	cm	kV	mA	Time	mAs	SID	Exposure Indicator
S							
M							
L							

Bontrager Textbook, 8th ed., p. 418.

Lateral Facial Bones

Evaluation Criteria

Anatomy Demonstrated:
- Superimposed facial bones, greater wings of sphenoid and sella turcica
- Region from orbital roofs to mentum demonstrated

Position:
- **No tilt;** evident by superimposition of orbital plates (roofs)
- **No rotation;** evident by superimposition of greater wings of sphenoid and mandibular rami

Exposure:
- Optimal density (brightness) and contrast to visualize facial structures
- Sharp bony margins; no motion

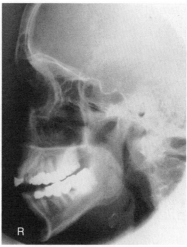

Fig. 8-22 Lateral facial bones.

Competency Check: _____
Technologist   Date

Skull, Facial Bones, and Paranasal Sinuses

8

Facial Bones—Parietoacanthial

(Waters and Modified Waters)

- 24 × 30 cm L.W. (10 × 12″) or 18 × 24 cm L.W. (8 × 10″)
- Grid

Position

Waters:

- Seated erect or prone on table
- Extend head resting on chin; place MML ⊥ to IR, which places the OML 37° to IR.
- Center IR to CR.

Modified Waters:

- OML is 55° to the plane of the IR, or line from junction of lips to EAM (LML) is ⊥ to IR.

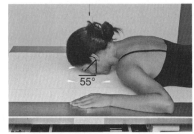

Fig. 8-23 PA Waters, OML 37°—CR and MML ⊥.

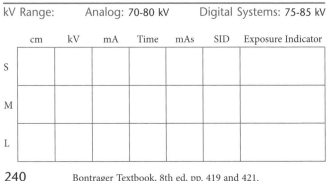

Fig. 8-24 PA modified Waters, OML 55°—CR and LML ⊥.

Central Ray: CR ⊥ to IR, to exit at acanthion (both projections)
SID: 40-44″ (102-113 cm)
Collimation: On four sides to area of facial bones
Respiration: Suspend during exposure.

kV Range:	Analog: 70-80 kV	Digital Systems: 75-85 kV

	cm	kV	mA	Time	mAs	SID	Exposure Indicator
S							
M							
L							

Parietoacanthial and Modified Parietoacanthial
(Waters and Modified Waters)

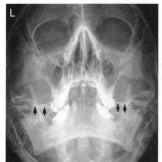

Fig. 8-25 PA Waters.

Competency Check: _____
                   Technologist   Date

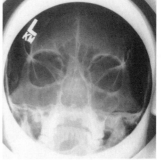

Fig. 8-26 PA modified Waters.

Competency Check: _____
                   Technologist   Date

Evaluation Criteria

Anatomy Demonstrated:

- **Waters:** Inferior orbital rims, maxillae, and nasal septum
- **Modified Waters:** Inferior orbital floors in profile (undistorted)

Position:

- **Waters:** Petrous ridges just inferior to floor of maxillary sinuses. **No rotation;** equal distance between orbits and lateral skull
- **Modified Waters:** Petrous ridges projected in lower $\frac{1}{2}$ of maxillary sinuses. **No rotation;** equal distance between orbits and lateral skull

Exposure:

- Optimal density (brightness) and contrast to visualize maxillary region and surrounding structures
- Sharp bony margins; no motion

Skull, Facial Bones, and Paranasal Sinuses

8

241

Facial Bones—PA Axial (Caldwell)

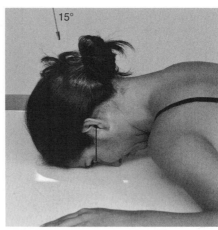

- 24 × 30 cm L.W. (10 × 12″) or 18 × 24 cm L.W. (8 × 10″)
- Grid

Position

- Seated erect or prone on table, MSP aligned to CR and to centerline of IR
- With forehead and nose resting on tabletop, adjust

Fig. 8-27 PA axial—15° Caldwell (OML ⊥); CR to exit at nasion.

head to place OML perpendicular to IR; ensure no rotation or tilt.
- Center IR to projected CR (to nasion).

Central Ray: CR 15° caudal to OML, centered to exit at nasion

Note: A 30° CR angle is required to project lower orbits below petrous ridges if this is an area of interest.

SID: 40-44″ (102-113 cm)

Collimation: On four sides to skull (facial bones) margins

Respiration: Suspend during exposure.

---

kV Range: Analog: 70-80 kV   Digital Systems: 75-85 kV

	cm	kV	mA	Time	mAs	SID	Exposure Indicator
S							
M							
L							

PA Axial (15° Caudad) Caldwell

Evaluation Criteria
Anatomy Demonstrated:
- **PA axial 15°:** Orbital rims, maxillae, nasal septum, and zygomatic arches

Position:
- **PA axial 15°:** Petrous ridges projected in lower $\frac{1}{3}$ of orbits. **No rotation;** equal distance between orbits and lateral skull margins

Exposure:
- Optimal density (brightness) and contrast to visualize maxillary region and orbital floor
- Sharp bony margins; no motion

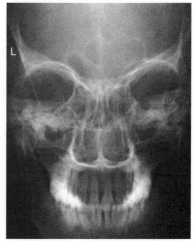

Fig. 8-28 PA axial Caldwell—15° caudad.

Competency Check: _____
　　　　　　　　　　Technologist　　　　Date

Skull, Facial Bones, and Paranasal Sinuses

8

Facial Bones—Trauma Series

Warning: With possible spine or severe head injuries, take all projections supine without moving head or without removing cervical collar if present.

Lateral (Horizontal Beam)

- 18 × 24 cm L.W. (8 × 10″)
- Grid, placed on edge against lateral cranium
- Ensure no rotation or tilt, MSP parallel to IR
- CR horizontal, to midway between outer canthus and EAM

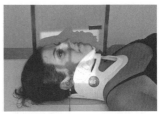

Fig. 8-29 Horizontal beam lateral—CR to midway between outer canthus and EAM.

Reverse Waters

- 18 × 24 cm L.W. (8 × 10″)
- Grid (Bucky), AEC—center field
- MSP aligned to CR and centerline of table or IR
- Ensure no rotation or tilt.
- CR parallel to MML
- CR centered to acanthion (CR angled cephalad as needed unless head can be tilted back if cervical injury has been ruled out).

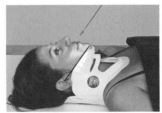

Fig. 8-30 Trauma reverse Waters—CR parallel to MML, centered to acanthion.

Reverse Modified Waters

- Same as reverse Waters except:
  - CR parallel to junction of lips-meatal line (LML), which is 18°-20° from MML
  - CR centered to acanthion

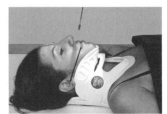

Fig. 8-31 Trauma reverse modified Waters—CR parallel to LML, centered to acanthion.

8

Optic Foramina—Parieto-orbital Oblique
(Rhese Method)

- 18 × 24 cm C.W. (8 × 10")
- Grid
- R and L sides taken for comparison
- AEC not recommended because of small body part

Position
- Seated erect or prone on table
- As a starting reference, adjust the head so the nose, cheek, and chin are touching the tabletop.
- Adjust the head so the AML is perpendicular to the IR, and the midsagittal plane is 53° to the IR (use angle indicator).
- Center IR to CR (to downside orbit).

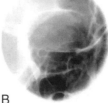

Fig. 8-32 A, Rhese oblique (right side).
B, Rhese oblique.
—AML and CR ⊥
—53° rotation of head from lateral

Central Ray: CR ⊥ to IR, to center of downside orbit
SID: 40-44" (102-113 cm)
Collimation: Closely collimate to 3-4" (8-10 cm) square.
Respiration: Suspend during exposure.

kV Range:	Analog: 70-80 kV			Digital Systems: 75-85 kV		
	cm	kV	mA	Time	mAs	SID	Exposure Indicator
S							
M							
L							

Bontrager Textbook, 8th ed, p. 427.

8

Zygomatic Arches—Bilateral
Submentovertex (SMV) Projection

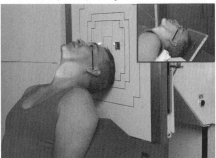

- 18 × 24 cm C.W. (8 × 10″)
- Nongrid or grid
- No AEC

Fig. 8-33 SMV, bilateral zygomatic arches, erect—CR ⊥ to IOML (nongrid may be preferred).

Position
- Seated erect or supine with head extended over end of table resting top of head against grid IR (may tilt table up slightly)
- Adjust IR and head to place IOML parallel to IR.
- Ensure no rotation or tilt.
- Center IR to CR.

Central Ray: CR angled as needed to be ⊥ to IOML, centered to midway between zygomatic arches (≈1.5″ or 4 cm inferior to mandibular symphysis)

SID: 40-44″ (102-113 cm)

Collimation: To include area of zygomatic arches

Respiration: Suspend during exposure.

kV Range:	Analog: 60-70 kV	Digital Systems: 70-80 kV

	cm	kV	mA	Time	mAs	SID	Exposure Indicator
S							
M							
L							

Bontrager Textbook, 8th ed, p. 424.

8

Zygomatic Arches—Tangential
(Oblique Inferosuperior Projection)

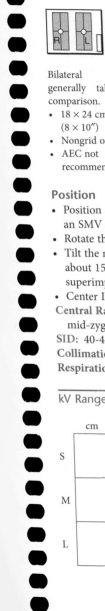

Bilateral arches generally taken for comparison.
- 18 × 24 cm C.W. (8 × 10″)
- Nongrid or grid
- AEC not recommended

Fig. 8-34 Tangential of left zygomatic arch—CR ⊥ to IOML, head tilted 15°, rotated 15°.

Position
- Position as for an SMV skull with the IOML parallel to the IR.
- Rotate the head ≈15° **toward** side being examined.
- Tilt the midsagittal plane with the chin **toward** the side of interest about 15° or as needed to free the zygomatic arch from superimposition by mandible or parietal bone.
- Center IR to CR.

Central Ray: CR angled if needed to be ⊥ to IOML, centered to mid-zygomatic arch

SID: 40-44″ (102-113 cm)

Collimation: Collimate closely to area of interest.

Respiration: Suspend during exposure.

kV Range:	Analog: 60-70 kV			Digital Systems: 70-80 kV		

	cm	kV	mA	Time	mAs	SID	Exposure Indicator
S							
M							
L							

Bontrager Textbook, 8th ed, p. 425.

Skull, Facial Bones, and Paranasal Sinuses

8

Submentovertex (SMV) and Oblique Tangential Zygomatic Arches

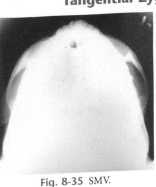

Fig. 8-35 SMV.

Competency Check: _____
　　　　　　　Technologist　　Date

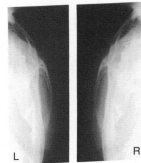

L　　　　　　　　　　　　R

Fig. 8-36 Oblique tangential.

Competency Check: _____
　　　　　　　Technologist　　Date

Evaluation Criteria

Anatomy Demonstrated:

- **SMV:** Bilateral zygomatic arches
- **Tangential:** Unilateral zygomatic arch

Position:

- **SMV:** Unobstructed view of bilateral arches. No rotation; symmetry of arches.
- **Oblique tangential:** Unilateral view of unobstructed arch. No superimposition of arch with parietal bone or mandible

Exposure:

- Optimal density (brightness) and contrast to visualize the zygomatic arches
- Sharp bony margins with soft tissue detail; no motion

Bilateral Zygomatic Arches—AP Axial
(Modified Towne)

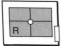

- 18 × 24 cm C.W. (8 × 10″)
- Grid
- AEC not recommended

Position

- Seated erect or supine on table, midsagittal plane aligned to midline of table or IR; ensure no rotation or tilt
- Depress chin to bring either the OML or the IOML perpendicular to IR.
- Center IR to projected CR.

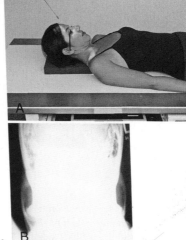

Fig. 8-37 **A**, AP axial—CR 37° to IOML. **B**, AP axial.

Skull, Facial Bones, and Paranasal Sinuses

Central Ray:

- CR 30° caudal to OML; or 37° to IOML
- CR 1″ (2.5 cm) superior to glabella to pass through level of midarches

SID: 40-44″ (102-113 cm)

Collimation: On four sides to area of bilateral arches

Respiration: Suspend during exposure.

kV Range:	Analog: 60-70 kV			Digital Systems: 70-80 kV			
	cm	kV	mA	Time	mAs	SID	Exposure Indicator
S							
M							
L							

Bontrager Textbook, 8th ed., p. 426.

Nasal Bones—Lateral

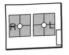

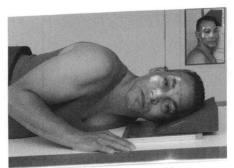

Bilateral projections generally taken for comparison.
- 18 × 24 cm C.W. (8 × 10″) (bilateral/ divided on same IR)
- Nongrid—detail screens

Fig. 8-38 Right lateral—nasal bones.

Position
- Seated erect or semiprone on table
- Center nasal bones to half of IR and to CR.
- Adjust head to bring IOML parallel to top and bottom edge of IR.
- Ensure a true lateral, IPL perpendicular to IR, and midsagittal plane parallel to IR.

Central Ray: CR ⊥ to IR, centered to ≈0.5″(1.25 cm) inferior to nasion

SID: 40-44″ (102-113 cm)

Collimation: Closely collimate to ≈4″ (10 cm) square.

Respiration: Suspend during exposure.

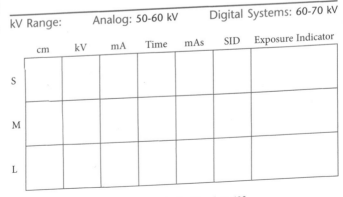

	cm	kV	mA	Time	mAs	SID	Exposure Indicator
S							
M							
L							

kV Range: Analog: 50-60 kV   Digital Systems: 60-70 kV

8

Bontrager Textbook, 8th ed, p. 422.

Lateral Nasal Bones

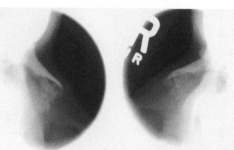

Fig. 8-39 Lateral nasal bones.

Competency Check: _____

Technologist   Date

Evaluation Criteria

Anatomy Demonstrated:
- Nasal bones with soft tissue structures
- Frontonasal suture to anterior nasal spine

Position:
- **No rotation;** complete profile of nasal bones
- Frontonasal suture to anterior nasal spine within collimation field

Exposure:
- Optimal density (brightness) and contrast to visualize nasal bones and surrounding soft tissue structures
- Sharp bony margins with soft tissue detail; no motion

8

Nasal Bones
Superoinferior Axial (Tangential) Projection

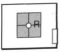

- 18 × 24 cm C.W. (8 × 10")
- Nongrid—detail screens

Position
- Seated erect at end of table or prone on table
- If prone, place supports under chest and under IR.
- Rest extended chin on IR, which should be perpendicular to GAL (glabelloalveolar line) and to CR.

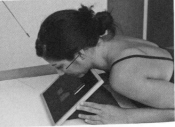

Fig. 8-40 Seated.

Central Ray: CR directed parallel to GAL, centered to nasion

SID: 40-44" (102-113 cm)

Collimation: Closely collimate to ≈4" (10 cm) square.

Respiration: Suspend during exposure.

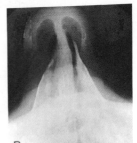

Fig. 8-41 Superoinferior.

kV Range: Analog: 50-60 kV   Digital Systems: 60-70 kV

cm	kV	mA	Time	mAs	SID	Exposure Indicator
S						
M						
L						

8

252

...tbook, 8th ed, p. 423.

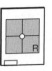

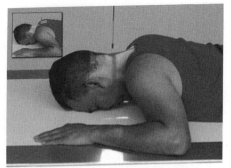

Skull, Facial Bones, and Paranasal Sinuses

- 18 × 24 cm L.W.
  (8 × 10″)
- Grid
- AEC not
  recommended

Fig. 8-42 PA mandible—CR and OML ⊥ to IR.)

Position
- Seated erect or
  prone on table,
  head aligned to
  centerline
- With forehead and nose resting on tabletop, adjust head to place
  OML ⊥ to IR.
- No rotation or tilt, midsagittal plane ⊥ to IR
- Center IR to CR (level of junction of lips).

Central Ray: CR ⊥ to IR, to exit at level of lips

Note: A CR angle of 20°-25° cephalad centered to exit at the
acanthion best demonstrates proximal rami and condyles.

SID: 40-44″ (102-113 cm)

Collimation: Collimate to area of mandible (square area).

Respiration: Suspend during exposure.

| kV Range: | Analog: 70-80 kV | | Digital Systems: 75-85 kV | | | | |

8

	cm	kV	mA	Time	mAs	SID	Exposure Indicator
S							
M							
L							

Mandible—Axiolateral Obliques

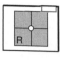

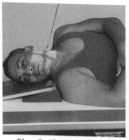

Fig. 8-43 Semisupine.

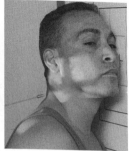

Fig. 8-44 Erect.
—CR 25° cephalad
—10°-15° head rotation for general survey (as shown above)
—0° head rotation for ramus
—30° head rotation for body
—45° head rotation for mentum

R and L sides generally taken for comparison unless contraindicated.

- 18 × 24 cm C.W. (8 × 10″)
- Grid or nongrid

Position

- Seated erect, semiprone, or semisupine, with support under shoulder and hip
- Extend chin, with side of interest against IR.
- Adjust head so IPL is perpendicular to IR, no tilt.
- Rotate head toward IR as determined by area of interest.

Central Ray: CR 25° cephalad to IPL, centered to downside midmandible (≈2″ or 5 cm below upside angle)

SID: 40-44″ (102-113 cm)

Collimation: To area of mandible (square area)

Respiration: Suspend during exposure.

kV Range: Analog: 70-80 kV Digital Systems: 75-80 kV

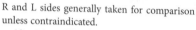

	cm	kV	mA	Time	mAs	SID	Exposure Indicator
S							
M							
L							

Bontrager Textbook, 8th ed, p. 428.

Mandible—Trauma Axiolateral Oblique

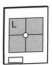

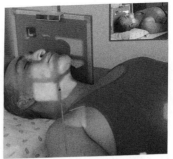

Fig. 8-45 Horizontal beam axiolateral—CR 30° cephalad from lateral, 5°-10° down.

For trauma patients unable to cooperate.
- 18 × 24 cm C.W. (8 × 10″)
- Grid or nongrid

Position
- Supine, no rotation of head, MSP ⊥ to TT
- IR on edge next to face, parallel to MSP with lower edge of IR ≈1″ (2.5 cm) below lower border of mandible
- Depress shoulders and elevate or extend chin if possible.

Note: May rotate head toward IR slightly (10°-15°) to better visualize body or mentum of mandible if this is area of interest.

Central Ray:
- CR horizontal beam, 30° cephalad (from lateral or IPL); angled down (posteriorly) 5°-10° to clear shoulder
- CR centered to ≈2″ (5 cm) distal to angle of mandible on side away from IR

SID: 40-44″ (102-113 cm)

Collimation: To area of mandible (square area)

Respiration: Suspend during exposure.

| kV Range: | Analog: 70-80 kV | | | | | Digital Systems: 75-80 kV |

	cm	kV	mA	Time	mAs	SID	Exposure Indicator
S							
M							
L							

Bontrager Textbook, 8th ed, pp. 428 and 598.

PA and Axiolateral Oblique Mandible

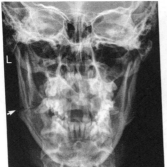

Fig. 8-46 PA mandible.

Competency Check: _____
                   Technologist   Date

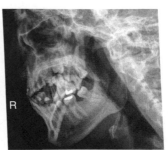

Fig. 8-47 Axiolateral oblique mandible.

Competency Check: _____
                   Technologist   Date

Evaluation Criteria

Anatomy Demonstrated:

- **PA:** Mandibular rami and lateral portion of body
- **Axiolateral:** Mandibular rami, condylar and coronoid processes, and body of near side

Position:

- **PA: No rotation** evident by symmetry of rami
- **Axiolateral:** Unobstructed view of mandibular rami, body, and mentum. No foreshortening of area of interest.

Exposure:

- Optimal density (brightness) and contrast to visualize mandibular area of interest
- Sharp bony margins; no motion

8

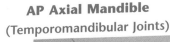

AP Axial Mandible
(Temporomandibular Joints)

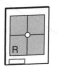

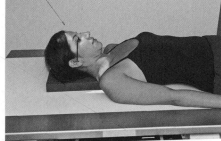

Fig. 8-48 AP axial, CR 35° to OML (CR centered for mandible).

- 18 × 24 cm L.W. (8 × 10″)
- Grid

Position
- Seated erect or supine on table, midsagittal plane centered to midline of table; ensure no rotation or tilt
- Depress chin to bring OML perpendicular to IR if possible (or bring IOML perpendicular and add 7° to CR angle).
- Center IR to projected CR.

Central Ray:
- CR 35° caudad to OML (42° to IOML)
- CR centered to glabella for mandible

Note: CR centered ≈2″ (5 cm) above glabella to pass through TMJs if TMJs are of primary interest.

SID: 40-44″ (102-113 cm)

Collimation: To include from TMJs to body of mandible

Respiration: Suspend during exposure.

Skull, Facial Bones, and Paranasal Sinuses

8

	cm	kV	mA	Time	mAs	SID	Exposure Indicator
kV Range:		Analog: 70-80 kV			Digital Systems: 75-85 kV		
S							
M							
L							

Temporomandibular Joints
Axiolateral Oblique (Modified Law Method)

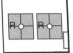

R and L sides for comparison in both open and closed mouth positions.

- 18 × 24 cm C.W. (8 × 10")
- Grid

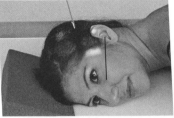

Fig. 8-49 Closed mouth.

Position

- Seated erect or semiprone on table, affected side down
- Adjust chin to place IOML parallel to top edge of IR.
- Anterior head (midsagittal plane) rotated 15° toward IR, no tilt, IPL remains perpendicular to IR
- Portion of IR being exposed centered to projected CR
- Second exposure in same position except with mouth fully open

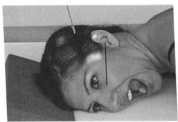

Fig. 8-50 Open mouth. —15° oblique (from lateral) and 15° CR (caudad)

Central Ray: CR 15° caudad, center to exit through downside TMJ (to enter 1.5" or 4 cm superior to upside EAM)

SID: 40-44" (102-113 cm)

Collimation: Collimate to 3-4" (8-10 cm) square.

Respiration: Suspend during exposure.

8

	cm	kV	mA	Time	mAs	SID	Exposure Indicator
S							
M							
L							

kV Range: Analog: 70-80 kV   Digital Systems: 75-85 kV

Temporomandibular Joints

Axiolateral (Schuller Method)

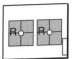

R and L sides for comparison in both open and closed mouth positions.
- 18 × 24 cm C.W. (8 × 10″)
- Grid

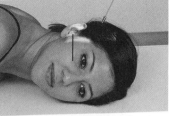

Fig. 8-51 Closed mouth.

Position
- Seated erect or semiprone, affected side down
- Adjust chin to place IOML parallel to top and bottom edges of IR, true lateral, no rotation or tilt of head.
- Portion of IR being exposed centered to projected CR
- Second exposure in same position except with mouth fully open

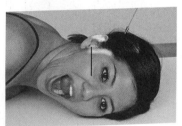

Fig. 8-52 Open mouth.
—25° caudad, 0° rotation

Central Ray: CR 25° caudad, center to exit through downside TMJ (to enter ≈2″ or 5 cm superior and 0.5″ or 1-2 cm anterior to upside EAM)

SID: 40-44″ (102-113 cm)

Collimation: Collimate to 3-4″ (8-10 cm) square.

Respiration: Suspend during exposure.

| kV Range: | Analog: 70-80 kV | | | | Digital Systems: 75-85 kV | |

	cm	kV	mA	Time	mAs	SID	Exposure Indicator
S							
M							
L							

Skull, Facial Bones, and Paranasal Sinuses

8

Axiolateral Oblique (Modified Law Method) and Axiolateral (Schuller method) TMJ Projections

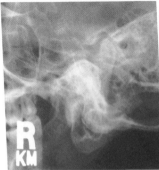

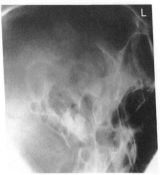

Fig. 8-53 Axiolateral oblique— closed mouth, downside TMJ shown in fossa (modified Law).

Competency Check: _____
                   Technologist   Date

Fig. 8-54 Axiolateral projection— open mouth; TMJ shown with condyle moved to anterior margin of fossa (Schuller).

Competency Check: _____
                   Technologist   Date

Note: Positioning routine would require both open and closed mouth of modified Law method, or both open and closed of Schuller method.

Evaluation Criteria

Anatomy Demonstrated:
- **Modified Law:** Bilateral, functional study of TMJ and fossa
- **Modified Schuller:** Bilateral, functional study of TMJ and fossa

8

Position:
- **Modified Law:** Unobstructed view of TMJ in both open and closed mouth positions (only closed mouth is shown)
- **Schuller:** Unobstructed view of TMJ in both open and closed mouth positions (only open mouth is shown)

Exposure:
- Optimal density (brightness) and contrast to visualize the TMJ and mandibular fossa
- Sharp bony margins; no motion

Lateral Paranasal Sinuses

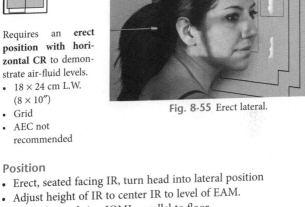
Fig. 8-55 Erect lateral.

Requires an **erect position with horizontal CR** to demonstrate air-fluid levels.

- 18 × 24 cm L.W. (8 × 10″)
- Grid
- AEC not recommended

Position

- Erect, seated facing IR, turn head into lateral position
- Adjust height of IR to center IR to level of EAM.
- Raise chin to bring IOML parallel to floor.
- No rotation, midsagittal plane parallel and IPL ⊥ to IR
- Center IR to CR.

Central Ray: CR horizontal to midpoint between EAM and outer canthus

SID: 40-44″ (102-113 cm)

Collimation: Collimate on four sides to area of sinuses.

Respiration: Suspend during exposure.

Skull, Facial Bones, and Paranasal Sinuses

8

		kV Range:	Analog: 65-75 kV		Digital Systems: 75-85 kV		
	cm	kV	mA	Time	mAs	SID	Exposure Indicator
S							
M							
L							

PA Paranasal Sinuses
(Caldwell Method)

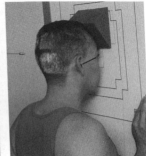

Requires an **erect position with horizontal CR** to demonstrate air-fluid levels.

- 18 × 24 cm L.W. (8 × 10″)
- Grid
- AEC not recommended

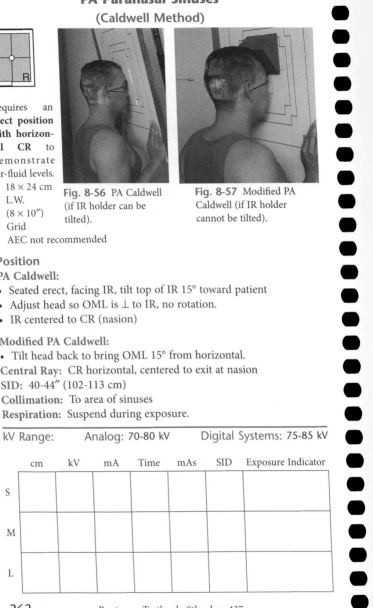

Fig. 8-56 PA Caldwell (if IR holder can be tilted).

Fig. 8-57 Modified PA Caldwell (if IR holder cannot be tilted).

Position
PA Caldwell:
- Seated erect, facing IR, tilt top of IR 15° toward patient
- Adjust head so OML is ⊥ to IR, no rotation.
- IR centered to CR (nasion)

Modified PA Caldwell:
- Tilt head back to bring OML 15° from horizontal.

Central Ray: CR horizontal, centered to exit at nasion
SID: 40-44″ (102-113 cm)
Collimation: To area of sinuses
Respiration: Suspend during exposure.

	kV Range:	Analog: 70-80 kV	Digital Systems: 75-85 kV

	cm	kV	mA	Time	mAs	SID	Exposure Indicator
S							
M							
L							

8

Bontrager Textbook, 8th ed, p. 437.

Lateral and PA Caldwell Sinuses

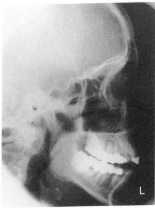

Fig. 8-58 Lateral sinuses.

Competency Check: _____
                  Technologist   Date

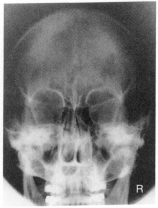

Fig. 8-59 PA axial (Caldwell) sinuses.

Competency Check: _____
                  Technologist   Date

Evaluation Criteria

Anatomy Demonstrated:
- **Lateral:** All paranasal sinuses demonstrated
- **PA Caldwell:** Frontal and anterior ethmoid sinuses

Position:
- **Lateral: No rotation or tilt;** superimposition of greater wings/ sphenoid, orbital roofs, and sella turcica
- **PA Caldwell:** Petrous ridges in lower $\frac{1}{3}$ of orbits. **No rotation;** equal distance between orbits and lateral skull

Exposure:
- Optimal density (brightness) and contrast to visualize the paranasal sinuses
- Sharp bony margins with soft tissue detail; no motion

Paranasal Sinuses
Parietoacanthial (Waters Method)

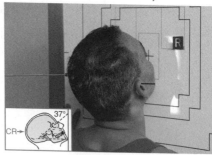

Fig. 8-60 PA erect Waters, MML ⊥, and CR horizontal.

Requires an **erect position with horizontal CR** to demonstrate air-fluid levels.

- 18 × 24 cm L.W. (8 × 10")
- Grid
- AEC not recommended

Position

- Seated erect, chin extended and touching IR holder
- Adjust height of IR to center IR to acanthion.
- Adjust MML perpendicular to IR (OML is 37° to IR).
- No rotation, midsagittal plane perpendicular to IR holder
- Center IR to CR.

Optional Open-Mouth Position

- Patient opens mouth wide to better visualize sphenoid sinuses through the open mouth

Central Ray: CR horizontal and ⊥ to IR, to exit at acanthion
SID: 40-44" (102-113 cm)
Collimation: Collimate on four sides to area of sinuses.
Respiration: Suspend during exposure.

kV Range:	Analog: 70-80 kV	Digital Systems: 75-85 kV

	cm	kV	mA	Time	mAs	SID	Exposure Indicator
S							
M							
L							

8

Bontrager Textbook, 8th ed, p. 438.

Paranasal Sinuses
Submentovertex (SMV)

Requires an **erect position with horizontal CR** to demonstrate air-fluid levels.

- 18 × 24 cm L.W. (8 × 10″)
- Grid
- AEC not recommended

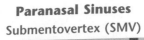

Fig. 8-61 SMV sinuses—CR ⊥ to IOML and IR.

Position
- Seated erect, leaning back in chair and extending head to rest top of head against IR holder
- Adjust head to place IOML as near parallel to plane of IR as possible; ensure no rotation or tilt.
- Center IR to CR.

Central Ray: CR horizontal and ⊥ to IOML, centered to midpoint between angles of mandible

SID: 40-44″ (102-113 cm)

Collimation: On four sides to area of sinuses

Respiration: Suspend during exposure.

	kV Range:	Analog: 70-80 kV			Digital Systems: 75-85 kV	
	cm	kV	mA	Time	mAs	SID	Exposure Indicator
S							
M							
L							

Parietoacanthial (Waters Method) Sinuses and Submentovertex (SMV)

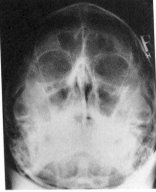

Fig. 8-62 PA (Waters) sinuses.

Competency Check: _____
Technologist   Date

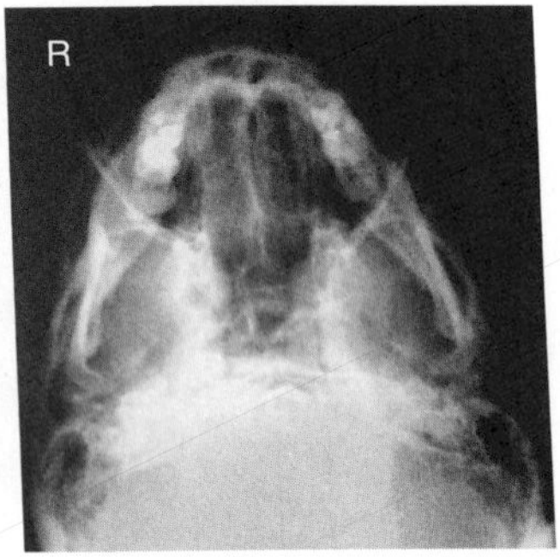

Fig. 8-63 SMV sinuses.

Competency Check: _____
Technologist   Date

Evaluation Criteria

Anatomy Demonstrated:

- **Waters:** Unobstructed view of maxillary sinuses
- **SMV:** Unobstructed view of sphenoid, maxillary, and ethmoid sinuses

Position:

- **Waters:** Petrous ridges just inferior to floor of maxillary sinuses. **No rotation;** equal distance between orbits and lateral skull
- **SMV:** Mandibular condyles projected anterior to petrous bone. **No rotation or tilt**; symmetry of petrous pyramids and equal distance between mandibular border and lateral skull

Exposure:

- Optimal density (brightness) and contrast to visualize the paranasal sinuses
- Sharp bony margins with soft tissue detail; no motion

Chapter 9

Abdomen and Common Contrast Media Procedures

9

(R) Routine, (S) Special

Abdomen and Common Contrast Media Procedures

Shielding and Positioning Landmarks

Gonadal Shielding

Male: Gonadal shields should be used on **all** males of reproductive age, with upper edge of shield placed at symphysis pubis unless it obscures essential anatomy.

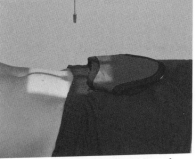

Fig. 9-1 Male gonadal shield (top of shield at symphysis pubis).

Females: Ovarian gonadal shields placed correctly may be used for abdomen examinations on females of reproductive age only **if** such shields do not obscure essential anatomy for that examination as determined by a radiologist (shielding is especially important for children).

Pregnancies Generally no radiographic procedures exposing the pelvic region should be performed during pregnancy without special instruction from a radiologist/physician.

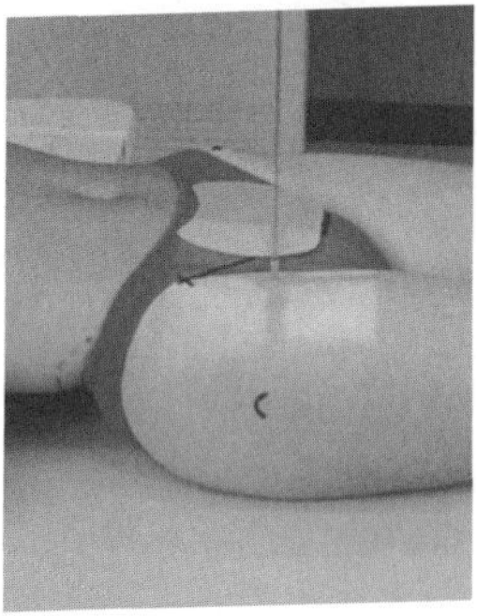

Fig. 9-2 Female ovarian shield (top of shield at or slightly above the level of ASIS, lower border just above symphysis pubis).

Topographic Positioning Landmarks

Certain positioning landmarks are essential for positioning the general abdomen and specific organs within the abdomen because the borders of these organs and the upper and lower margins of the general abdomen itself are not visible from the exterior.

Abdominal borders and organ locations, however, can be determined by certain landmarks, which can be located by gentle palpation with the fingertips, being careful of painful or sensitive areas. (The patient should be informed of the purpose for this before beginning the palpation process.)

Barium Distribution and Body Positions

The air-barium distribution within the stomach and large intestine changes with various body positions. By knowing these distribution patterns, one can determine in which body position a radiograph was taken. Air always rises to the highest levels, and the heavy barium settles to the lowest levels (air is black, barium is white).

Stomach

The fundus is located more posteriorly; therefore in the supine position it would be the lowest portion of the stomach and would be filled with barium.

In both prone and erect positions, the fundus would be filled with air as seen on the drawings below, with a straight air-barium line on the erect.

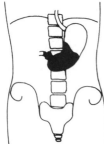

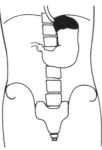

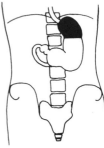

Fig. 9-3 Supine (barium in fundus).

Fig. 9-4 Prone (barium in body and pylorus).

Fig. 9-5 Erect (straight-line barium-air level).
Barium = white
Air = black

Large Intestine

The ascending and descending portions are located more posteriorly, and thus more of these parts in general would be filled with barium (white) in the **supine position** and with air (black) in the **prone position.**

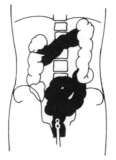

Fig. 9-6 Supine.

Fig. 9-7 Prone.

Note: This much separation of barium and air occurs generally only with double-contrast barium-air studies.

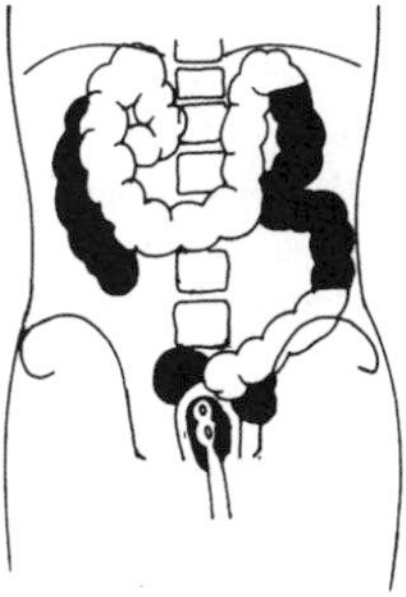

Air-fluid levels would be seen in the **erect position** in which the air would rise to the highest position in each of the various sections of the large intestine, as shown in the accompanying figure.

Right and left decubitus projections (not shown on these drawings) also would demonstrate air-fluid levels, with air again rising to the highest portions.

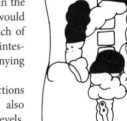

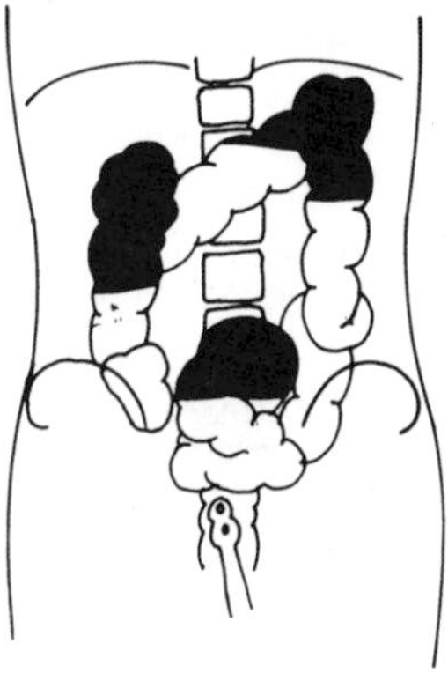

Fig. 9-8 Erect.

9

AP Abdomen (KUB)

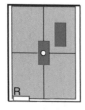

- 35 × 43 cm L.W.
  (14 × 17″)
- Grid

Fig. 9-9 KUB abdomen.

Position

- Supine, legs extended, arms at sides
- Midsagittal plane aligned and centered to centerline
- Ensure no rotation (ASISs equal distance from tabletop)
- Center of IR to level of iliac crests, ensuring that upper margin of symphysis pubis is included on lower IR margin. (A large hypersthenic patient may require that the IR be placed crosswise with a second IR centered higher.)

Central Ray: CR ⊥, to center of IR (level of iliac crests)
SID: 40-44″ (102-113 cm)
Collimation: To abdomen or IR borders
Respiration: Expose at end of expiration.

---

kV Range: Analog and Digital Systems*: 70-80 kV
*Recommended kV ranges are identical for analog and digital systems to prevent overpenetration of small calculi in the abdomen.

	cm	kV	mA	Time	mAs	SID	Exposure Indicator
S							
M							
L							

9

Erect AP Abdomen

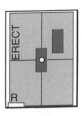

- 35 × 43 cm L.W. (14 × 17")
- Grid
- Erect marker

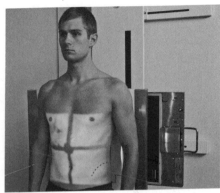

Fig. 9-10 Erect AP (include diaphragm).

Position
- Erect, back against table, arms at sides
- Midsagittal plane aligned and centered to centerline
- Ensure no rotation
- Center of IR approximately 2-3" (5-6.5 cm) above iliac crest to include diaphragm

Central Ray: CR horizontal, to center of IR (2-3" [5-6.5 cm] above iliac crest)

SID: 40-44" (102-113 cm)

Collimation: To include abdomen and diaphragm

Respiration: Expose at end of expiration.

Abdomen and Common Contrast Media Procedures

kV Range:			Analog and Digital Systems: 70-80 kV				
	cm	kV	mA	Time	mAs	SID	Exposure Indicator
S							
M							
L							

AP Supine and AP Erect Abdomen

Evaluation Criteria

Anatomy Demonstrated:

- **AP supine:** Outline of liver, spleen, psoas muscles, and kidneys to include symphysis pubis lower abdomen
- **AP erect:** Bilateral diaphragm and significant portion of lower abdomen

Position:

- **AP supine and erect:** No rotation; symmetry of iliac wings and outer, lower rib margins

Exposure:

- Optimal density (brightness) and contrast to visualize psoas muscles and lumbar transverse processes
- Air-fluid levels seen if present
- Liver margins and kidneys visible on patients of average size; no motion

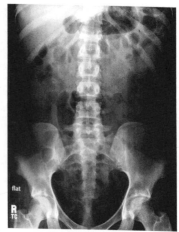

Fig. 9-11 AP supine.

Competency Check: _____
Technologist   Date

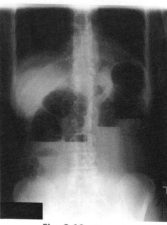

Fig. 9-12 AP erect.

Competency Check: _____
Technologist   Date

Abdomen
Lateral Decubitus (AP)

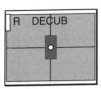

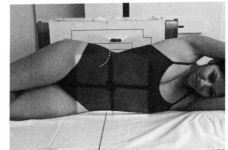

- 35 × 43 cm C.W. (14 × 17″)
- Grid
- Decubitus marker
- Arrow marker to include upside

Fig. 9-13 Left lateral decubitus (AP).

- Patient should be on side **a minimum of 5 minutes** before exposure; **10 to 20 minutes is preferred.**

Position

- Lock wheels of stretcher
- Patient on side (on decubitus board or support to elevate downside abdomen), knees partially flexed, arms up near head
- Adjust patient and stretcher so center of IR and table (and CR) is approximately 2″ (5 cm) above level of iliac crest (to include diaphragm)
- Adjust height of IR to ensure that upside of abdomen is included for possible free air

Central Ray: CR horizontal, to center of IR
SID: 40-44″ (102-113 cm)
Collimation: Entire abdomen and diaphragm
Respiration: Expose at end of expiration.

| kV Range: | | | Analog and Digital Systems: 70-80 kV | | | | |

	cm	kV	mA	Time	mAs	SID	Exposure Indicator
S							
M							
L							

Abdomen and Common Contrast Media Procedures

9

Abdomen

Dorsal Decubitus (Lateral)

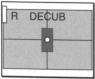

- 35 × 43 cm C.W. (14 × 17″)
- Grid
- Include decubitus marker

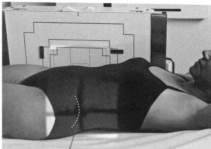

Fig. 9-14 Dorsal decubitus (R lateral).

Position

- Patient supine (on decubitus board or support to elevate posterior abdomen), side against table, arms above head
- Secure stretcher (lock wheels)
- Center of IR and table (and CR) at level of iliac crest (2″ above iliac crest to include diaphragm)
- Adjust height of IR to align midcoronal plane to centerline of IR

Central Ray: CR horizontal, to center of IR

SID: 40-44″ (102-113 cm)

Collimation: To abdomen or IR borders

Respiration: Expose at end of expiration.

kV Range:				Analog and Digital Systems: 70-80 kV			
	cm	kV	mA	Time	mAs	SID	Exposure Indicator
S							
M							
L							

Bontrager Textbook, 8th ed, p. 120.

Lateral and Dorsal Decubitus Abdomen

Evaluation Criteria

Anatomy Demonstrated:

- **Lateral decubitus:** Abdomen visualized to include air-filled stomach and bowel and upside diaphragm

- **Dorsal decubitus:** Abdomen visualized to include bilateral diaphragm

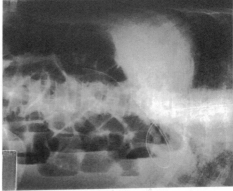

Fig. 9-15 Lateral decubitus.

Competency Check: _____
                    Technologist   Date

Position:

- **Lateral decubitus:** **No rotation;** symmetry of iliac wings and spine straight

- **Dorsal decubitus:** **No rotation;** symmetry of

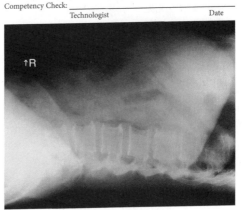

Fig. 9-16 Dorsal decubitus.

Competency Check: _____
                    Technologist   Date

iliac wings and diaphragm. Intervertebral joint spaces and vertebral bodies should be visible.

Exposure:

- Optimal density (brightness) and contrast to visualize soft tissue structures and lumbar spine
- Soft tissue structures and any intraperitoneal air demonstrated on patients of average size; no motion

AP Pediatric Abdomen (KUB)

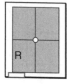

- 18 × 24, 24 × 30, or 30 × 35 cm L.W.
- Screen <10 cm, grid >10 cm

Fig. 9-17 Child AP abdomen (KUB).

Position (Infant)

- Immobilize arms above head (use stockinette, Ace bandage, tape, or sandbags).
- Immobilize legs with Ace bandage or tape and sandbags.
- Center IR to CR.
- Shield gonads if possible.

Parental Assistance for Infant: Use only if necessary. Supply with lead apron and gloves, and have parent hold arms above head with one hand and legs with other hand, preventing rotation.

Central Ray: Newborns to 1 year old: CR to 1″ or 2.5 cm above umbilicus. Older child: CR to level of umbilicus.

SID: 40-44″ (102-113 cm)

Collimation: On four sides to abdominal borders

Respiration: Expose on expiration or when abdomen has least movement. If crying, time exposures at full expiration.

kV Range:	Analog: 65-75 kV	Digital Systems: 70-80 kV

	cm	kV	mA	Time	mAs	SID	Exposure Indicator
S							
M							
L							

9

Bontrager Textbook, 8th ed, p. 644.

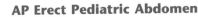

AP Erect Pediatric Abdomen

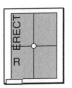

- 18 × 24, 24 × 30, or 30 × 35 cm L.W.
- Screen <10 cm, Grid >10 cm

Position
- Patient seated, legs through openings
- Arms above head, side body clamps firmly in place
- Lead shield at level of symphysis pubis, center IR to CR

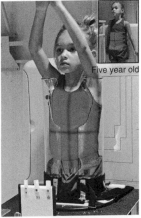

Fig. 9-18 Utilizing Pigg-O-Stat.

Parental Assistance: If necessary, have parent hold arms overhead with one hand, and with other hand hold legs to prevent rotation of pelvis or thorax (provide with lead apron and gloves).

Central Ray: Newborn to 1 year old: CR to 1″ (2.5 cm) above umbilicus. Older child: CR to level of umbilicus.

SID: 40-44″ (102-113 cm)

Collimation: On four sides to abdominal borders

Respiration: Expose on expiration, or during least movement.

kV Range:	Analog: 65-75 kV			Digital Systems: 70-80 kV		
	cm	kV	mA	Time	mAs	SID	Exposure Indicator
S							
M							
L							

Abdomen and Common Contrast Media Procedures

9

AP Supine and Erect Pediatric Abdomen

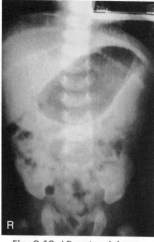

Fig. 9-19 AP supine abdomen.

Competency Check: _____
                            Technologist   Date

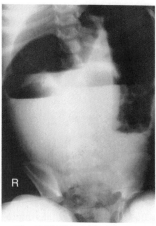

Fig. 9-20 Erect AP abdomen.

Competency Check: _____
                            Technologist   Date

Evaluation Criteria
Anatomy Demonstrated:

- **AP supine and erect:** Soft tissue and gas-filled structures; air-fluid levels on erect

Position:
- **AP supine and erect:** Diaphragm to symphysis pubis included if possible

Exposure:
- Optimal density (brightness) and contrast to visualize soft tissue structures and skeletal structures; no motion

9

Esophagogram—RAO

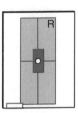

- 35 × 43 cm L.W. (14 × 17")
- Grid

Position
- Recumbent or erect, recumbent preferred for better filling of esophagus
- Rotate 35°-40° from prone position onto right side, right arm down, left arm up; hold cup with left hand, straw in mouth.

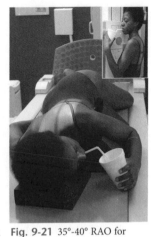

Fig. 9-21 35°-40° RAO for esophagus (barium swallow).

- Center thorax to centerline.
- Top of IR ≈2" (5 cm) above level of shoulder

Central Ray: CR ⊥, to center of IR (≈3" or 7 cm distal to jugular notch at T6 level)

SID: 40-44" (102-113 cm)

Collimation: To area of interest (≈5-6" [12-15 cm] wide)

Respiration: With thin barium, expose while swallowing (after 3 or 4 swallows). With thick barium, expose immediately after swallowing (while holding breath).

		Analog and Digital Systems: 100-125 kV
kV Range:		

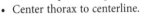

	cm	kV	mA	Time	mAs	SID	Exposure Indicator
S							
M							
L							

Bontrager Textbook, 8th ed, p. 478.

Esophagogram—Lateral

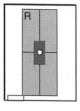

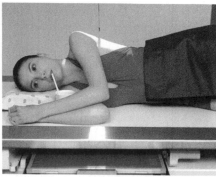

Fig. 9-22 R lateral esophagogram (barium swallow) in "swimmer's" position.

- 35 × 43 cm L.W. (14 × 17″)
- Grid

Position

- Recumbent or erect, recumbent preferred
- Right lateral position, right arm and shoulder up and forward (holding cup), left arm and shoulder down and back
- Center midcoronal plane to centerline.
- Top of IR ≈2″ (5 cm) above top of shoulder

Central Ray: CR ⊥, to center of IR (≈3″ or 7 cm distal to jugular notch at T6 level)

SID: 40-44″ (102-113 cm) or 72″ (183 cm) if performed erect

Collimation: To area of interest (5-6″ [12-15 cm] wide)

Respiration: With thin barium, expose while swallowing (after 3 or 4 swallows). With thick barium, expose immediately after swallowing, while holding breath.

	cm	kV	mA	Time	mAs	SID	Exposure Indicator
S							
M							
L							

kV Range: Analog and Digital Systems: 100-125 kV

RAO and Lateral Esophagogram

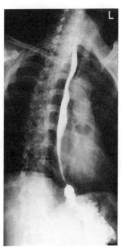

Fig. 9-23 RAO esophagogram.

Competency Check: _____
Technologist   Date

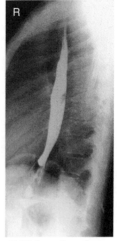

Fig. 9-24 Lateral esophagogram.

Competency Check: _____
Technologist   Date

Evaluation Criteria

Anatomy Demonstrated:
- **RAO:** Esophagus visible between vertebral column and heart
- **Lateral:** Entire esophagus seen between thoracic spine and heart

Position:
- **RAO:** Entire esophagus lined with contrast media and not superimposed over spine
- **Lateral:** No rotation; superimposition of posterior ribs, entire esophagus lined with contrast media

Exposure:
- Optimal density (brightness) and contrast to visualize borders of contrast-filled esophagus
- Sharp structural margins; no motion

Esophagogram—AP (PA)

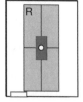

- 35 × 43 cm L.W.
  (14 × 17″)
- Grid

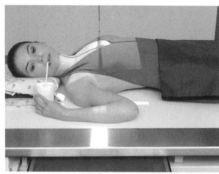

Fig. 9-25 AP esophagogram (barium swallow).

Position

- Supine or erect, supine preferred (may be taken PA if erect)
- Center patient to centerline.
- Top of IR ≈2″ (5 cm) above top of shoulder
- Left arm at side, holding cup with right hand, straw in mouth

Central Ray: CR ⊥, to center of IR (≈3″ or 7 cm distal to jugular notch at T6)

SID: 40-44″ (102-113 cm) or 72″ (183 cm) if performed erect

Collimation: To area of interest (5-6″ [12-15 cm] wide)

Respiration: With thin barium, expose while swallowing (after 3 or 4 swallows). With thick barium, expose immediately after swallowing, while holding breath.

Abdomen and Common Contrast Media Procedures

9

kV Range:		Analog and Digital Systems: 100-125 kV				
	cm	kV	mA	Time	mAs	SID	Exposure Indicator
S							
M							
L							

Bontrager Textbook, 8th ed, p. 480.

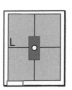

- 35 × 43 cm L.W. (14 × 17″), 30 × 35 cm (11 × 14″), or 24 × 30 cm (10 × 12″), L.W.
- Grid

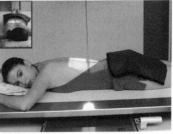

Fig. 9-26 PA upper GI (stomach).

Position

- Prone, arms up beside head
- Align and center patient and IR to CR.

Central Ray: CR ⊥, centered as follows:

Sthenic:
Center ≈1″ (2.5 cm) above lower rib margin (level of L1) and ≈1″ (2.5 cm) to left of vertebral column

Hypersthenic:
Center 2″ (5 cm) higher

Asthenic:
Center ≈2″ (5 cm) lower and nearer midline

SID: 40-44″ (102-113 cm)

Collimation: To outer margins of IR or to area of interest

Respiration: Expose at end of expiration.

kV Range:	Analog and Digital Systems: 100-125 kV
	90-100 kV for Double-Contrast Study
	80-90 kV (Water-Soluble Contrast Media)

	cm	kV	mA	Time	mAs	SID	Exposure Indicator
S							
M							
L							

Abdomen and Common Contrast Media Procedures

9

Upper GI—RAO

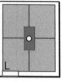

- 30 × 35 cm (11 × 14″) or 24 × 30 cm (10 × 12″) L.W.
- Grid

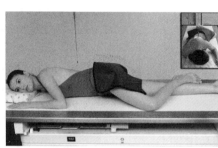

Fig. 9-27 40°-70° RAO, upper GI (stomach).

Position

- Semiprone, rotate 40°-70° from prone toward right side
- Right arm down, left arm up, partially flex left hip and knee
- Align and center patient to CR

Central Ray: CR ⊥, to duodenal bulb region

Sthenic:

Center ≈1″ (2.5 cm) above lower ribs and midway between vertebrae and left lateral abdominal border, 45°-55° oblique from prone

Hypersthenic:

Center 1-2″ (3-5 cm) higher, ≈70° oblique

Asthenic:

Center ≈2″ (5 cm) lower, ≈40° oblique

SID: 40-44″ (102-113 cm)

Collimation: To outer margins of IR or to area of interest

Respiration: Expose at end of expiration.

kV Range:	Analog and Digital Systems: 100-125 kV
	90-100 kV for Double-Contrast Study
	80-90 kV (Water-Soluble Contrast Media)

	cm	kV	mA	Time	mAs	SID	Exposure Indicator
S							
M							
L							

Bontrager Textbook, 8th ed, p. 482.

PA and RAO Upper GI

Evaluation Criteria
Anatomy Demonstrated:
- **PA:** Entire stomach and duodenum
- **RAO:** Entire stomach and C-loop of duodenum

Position:
- **PA:** Body and pylorus are barium-filled; body and pylorus are centered
- **RAO:** Pylorus and duodenal bulb barium-filled; duodenal bulb in profile

Exposure:
- Optimal density (brightness) and contrast to visualize gastric folds without overexposing other structures
- Sharp structural margins; no motion

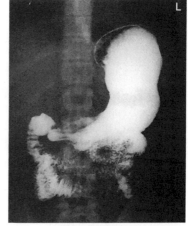

Fig. 9-28 PA.

Competency Check: _____
                    Technologist   Date

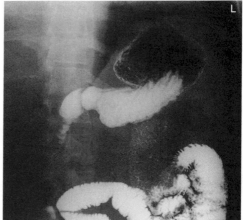

Fig. 9-29 RAO.

Competency Check: _____
                    Technologist   Date

Abdomen and Common Contrast Media Procedures

9

287

Upper GI—Lateral

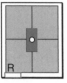

- 30 × 35 cm L.W. (11 × 14″) or 24 × 30 cm L.W. (10 × 12″)
- Grid

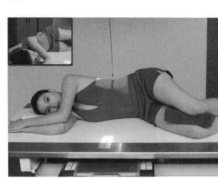

Fig. 9-30 Right lateral upper GI (stomach).

Position
- Patient on right side, arms up, hips and knees partially flexed
- Align and center patient and IR to CR.

Central Ray: CR ⊥, to region of pylorus as follows:

Sthenic:
Center to margin of ribs, and to anterior $1/3$ of abdomen

Hypersthenic:
Center ≈2″ (5 cm) higher

Asthenic:
Center ≈2″ (5 cm) lower
SID: 40-44″ (102-113 cm)
Collimation: To outer margins of IR or to area of interest
Respiration: Expose at end of expiration.

kV Range:	Analog and Digital Systems: 100-125 kV
	90-100 kV for Double-Contrast Study
	80-90 kV (Water-Soluble Contrast Media)

	cm	kV	mA	Time	mAs	SID	Exposure Indicator
S							
M							
L							

9

Bontrager Textbook, 8th ed, p. 484.

Upper GI—AP

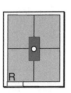

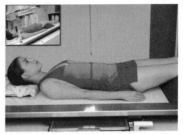

- 30 × 35 cm L.W. (11 × 14") or
  24 × 30 cm L.W. (10 × 12")
- Grid

Fig. 9-31 AP supine Trendelenburg, upper GI (stomach) (Trendelenburg position best demonstrates hiatal hernia).

Position
- Supine, arms at side
- Align and center patient and IR to CR.

Central Ray: CR ⊥, centered to 2.5-5 cm (1-2") to left of MSP

Sthenic:
Center to level of L1 (midway between xiphoid process and level of lower lateral ribs)

Hypersthenic:
Center ≈2.5 cm (1") higher

Asthenic:
Center ≈5 cm (2") lower and nearer midline
SID: 40-44" (102-113 cm)
Collimation: To outer IR margins or to area of interest
Respiration: Expose at end of expiration.

---

kV Range:	Analog and Digital Systems: 100-125 kV
	90-100 kV for Double-Contrast Study
	80-90 kV (Water-Soluble Contrast Media)

	cm	kV	mA	Time	mAs	SID	Exposure Indicator
S							
M							
L							

Abdomen and Common Contrast Media Procedures

9

Lateral and AP Upper GI

Abdomen and Common Contrast Media Procedures

9

Evaluation Criteria

Anatomy Demonstrated:

- **Lateral:** Entire stomach and duodenum and retrogastric space demonstrated
- **AP:** Entire stomach and C-loop of duodenum; diaphragm included to r/o hiatal hernia

Position:

- **Lateral:** Pylorus and C-loop of duodenum demonstrated. **No rotation;** evident by aligned vertebral bodies
- **AP:** Fundus barium-filled and centered

Exposure:

- Optimal density (brightness) and contrast to visualize gastric folds without overexposing other structures
- Sharp structural margins; no motion

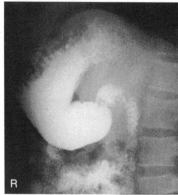

Fig. 9-32 Lateral upper GI.

Competency Check: _____
Technologist   Date

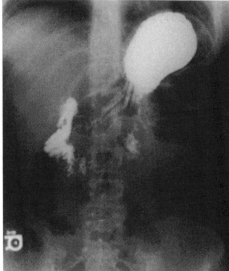

Fig. 9-33 AP upper GI.

Competency Check: _____
Technologist   Date

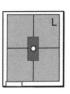

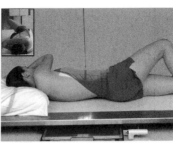

- 30 × 35 cm L.W. (11 × 14″) or
  24 × 30 cm L.W. (10 × 12″)
- Grid

Position

Fig. 9-34 30°-60° LPO, upper GI (stomach).

- Semisupine, 30°-60°
  oblique,* left side down, partially flex right knee
- Center patient and IR to CR

Central Ray: CR ⊥, centered to left half of abdomen

*More rotation for hypersthenic patients

Sthenic:

Center to L1 (midway between xiphoid process and level of lower lateral ribs), 45° oblique

Hypersthenic:

Center 2.5 cm (1″) higher, 60° oblique

Asthenic:

≈5 cm (2″) lower and nearer midline, 30°

SID: 40-44″ (102-113 cm)

Collimation: To outer IR margins or to area of interest

Respiration: Expose at end of expiration.

kV Range:	Analog and Digital Systems: 100-125 kV
	90-100 kV for Double-Contrast Study
	80-90 kV (Water-Soluble Contrast Media)

	cm	kV	mA	Time	mAs	SID	Exposure Indicator
S							
M							
L							

Abdomen and Common Contrast Media Procedures

9

LPO Upper GI

Evaluation Criteria
Anatomy Demonstrated:

- Entire stomach and duodenum; unobstructed view of duodenal bulb

Position:

- Fundus is barium-filled; gas-filled duodenal bulb seen for double-contrast study
- Duodenal bulb in profile

Exposure:

- Optimal density (brightness) and contrast to visualize gastric folds without overexposing other structures
- Sharp structural and gastric organ margins; no motion

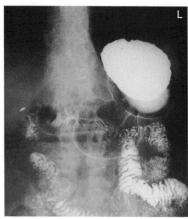

Fig. 9-35 LPO upper GI.

Competency Check: _____
                    Technologist   Date

Small Bowel Series—PA

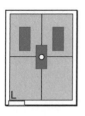

A common routine includes images at 15- or 30-minute intervals until barium reaches ileocecal valve.

- 35 × 43 cm L.W. (14 × 17″)
- Grid

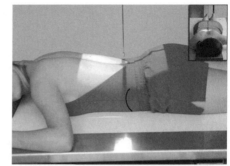

Fig. 9-36 PA small bowel (15 or 30 min).

Position

- Prone preferred (may be taken AP supine if necessary)
- MSP aligned to centerline; no rotation
- Center patient and IR to iliac crest (center higher on early IRs).

Central Ray: CR ⊥, to center of IR, ≈2″ (5 cm) above level of iliac crest for early IRs (15 or 30 min), and at iliac crest for later images

SID: 40-44″ (102-113 cm)

Collimation: To outer margins of IR or to area of interest

Respiration: Expose at end of full expiration.

kV Range:			Analog and Digital Systems: 100-125 kV			
	cm	kV	mA	Time	mAs	SID	Exposure Indicator
S							
M							
L							

9

Barium Enema—PA or AP

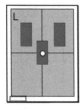

- 35 × 43 cm L.W. (14 × 17″)
- Grid

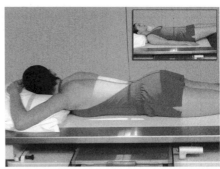

Fig. 9-37 PA barium enema.

Position

- Patient prone (PA) or supine (AP); work quickly
- Patient aligned and centered to centerline; no rotation
- Center IR to level of iliac crest (see *Note*).

Central Ray: CR ⊥, to center of IR, at level of iliac crest

Note: For large or hypersthenic patients, the use of two IRs may be necessary, placed crosswise if the entire colon is to be included (one centered for lower abdomen and one for upper abdomen).

SID: 40-44″ (102-113 cm)

Collimation: To outer IR borders or to area of interest

Respiration: Expose at full expiration.

---

kV Range:

Analog and Digital Systems:
100-125 kV (Single Contrast)
90-100 kV (Double Contrast)
80-90 kV (Water-Soluble Contrast Media)

	cm	kV	mA	Time	mAs	SID	Exposure Indicator
S							
M							
L							

9

294 Bontrager Textbook, 8th ed, p. 515.

PA (AP) Barium Enema

Evaluation Criteria
Anatomy Demonstrated:
- Entire large intestine demonstrated, including left colic flexure and rectum

Position:
- Transverse colon primarily filled with barium (PA) and gas-filled with AP
- **No rotation;** evident by symmetry of ala of ilium and lumbar vertebra

Exposure:
- Optimal density (brightness) and contrast to visualize mucosa without overexposing other structures
- Sharp structural margins; no motion

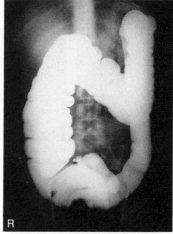

Fig. 9-38 PA single-contrast BE.

Competency Check: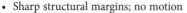

Technologist   Date

9

Barium Enema—RAO and LAO

(or RPO and LPO)

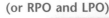

Abdomen and Common Contrast Media Procedures

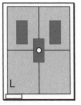

L

Both right and left oblique projections are commonly taken.

- 35 × 43 cm L.W. (14 × 17″)
- Grid

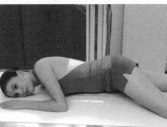

Fig. 9-39 35°-45° RAO barium enema.

Position

- Semiprone (PA) or semisupine (AP), rotated 35°-45°
- Align and center abdomen to centerline.
- IR centered to level of iliac crest (include rectal area)

Central Ray: CR ⊥ to center of IR (at level of iliac crest)

Note: Many patients require a second IR centered ≈2″ (5 cm) higher if the left colic flexure is to be included—most important on **LAO** or **RPO** (determine departmental routine).

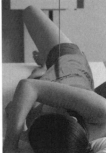

Fig. 9-40 35°-45° LPO.

SID: 40-44″ (102-113 cm)

Collimation: To outer IR borders or to area of interest

Respiration: Expose at expiration.

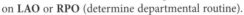

kV Range:				Analog and Digital Systems:

100-125 kV (Single Contrast)
90-100 kV (Double Contrast)
80-90 kV (Water-Soluble Contrast Media)

	cm	kV	mA	Time	mAs	SID	Exposure Indicator
S							
M							
L							

9

Bontrager Textbook, 8th ed, pp. 516 and 517.

Oblique Barium Enema

Evaluation Criteria

Anatomy Demonstrated:
- **LPO/RAO:** Right colic flexure, ascending, and sigmoid colon
- **RPO/LAO:** Left colic flexure and descending colon

Position:
- **LPO/RAO:** Right colic flexure and ascending colon in profile
- **RPO/LAO:** Left colic flexure in profile, and descending colon in profile

Exposure:
- Appropriate technique (brightness) to visualize mucosa without overexposing other structures
- Sharp structural margins; no motion

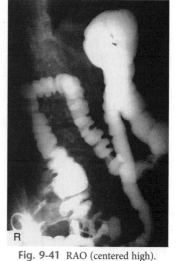

Fig. 9-41 RAO (centered high).

Competency Check: _____
Technologist   Date

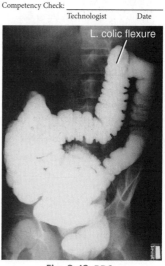

L. colic flexure

Fig. 9-42 RPO.

Competency Check: _____
Technologist   Date

297

Barium Enema—Lateral Rectum
(Ventral Decubitus)

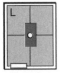

Alternative ventral decubitus projection is often performed for double-contrast studies.

- 24 × 30 cm L.W. (10 × 12″) or 30 × 35 cm L.W. (11 × 14″)
- Grid
- Compensating filter for ventral decubitus lateral

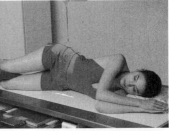
Fig. 9-43 Left lateral for rectum.

Position

- Recumbent in true lateral position; work quickly
- Center midaxillary plane to centerline, with knees and hips partially flexed
- Center patient and IR to CR.

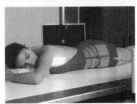
Fig. 9-44 Ventral decubitus lateral rectum (alternate projection with double-contrast examination).

Central Ray: CR ⊥, to level of ASIS, centered to midcoronal plane (midway between ASIS and posterior sacrum). CR is **horizontal** for ventral decubitus.

SID: 40-44″ (102-113 cm)

Collimation: To outer IR borders or to area of interest

Respiration: Expose at expiration.

---

kV Range: Analog and Digital Systems:
100-125 kV (Single Contrast) 90-100 kV (Double Contrast)
80-90 kV (Water-Soluble Contrast Media)

	cm	kV	mA	Time	mAs	SID	Exposure Indicator
S							
M							
L							

Barium Enema—Lateral Decubitus

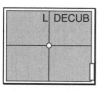

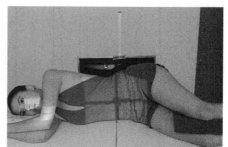

Fig. 9-45 Right lateral decubitus (AP).

Both right and left lateral decubitus are commonly taken as part of a double-contrast series.

- 35 × 43 cm L.W. to patient (14 × 17″)
- Grid (portable grid or Bucky)
- Compensating filter placed on upside of abdomen

Position

- Patient on side, arms up, knees partially flexed, back against grid cassette or table
- MSP aligned and centered to centerline of IR (and CR); no rotation (lock wheels if stretcher is used)
- IR centered to level of iliac crest

Central Ray: CR horizontal to center of IR (to level of iliac crest at midsagittal plane)

SID: 40-44″ (102-113 cm)

Collimation: To outer IR borders or to area of interest

Respiration: Expose at full expiration.

kV Range:	Analog and Digital Systems: 90-100 kV (Double-Contrast Study)

	cm	kV	mA	Time	mAs	SID	Exposure Indicator
S							
M							
L							

Abdomen and Common Contrast Media Procedures

9

Barium Enema—AP (PA)
Axial (Butterfly Position)

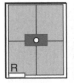

- 30 × 35 cm L.W. (11 × 14″) or 24 × 30 cm L.W. (10 × 12″)
- Grid

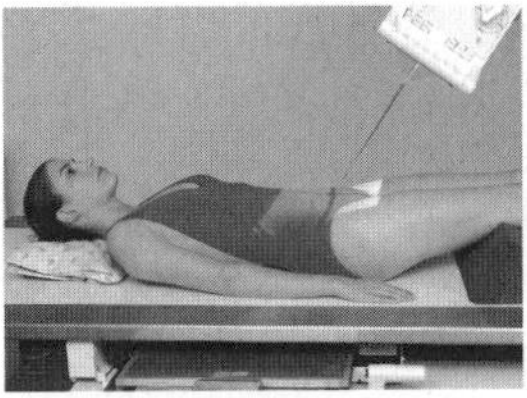

Fig. 9-46 AP—CR 30°-45° cephalad.

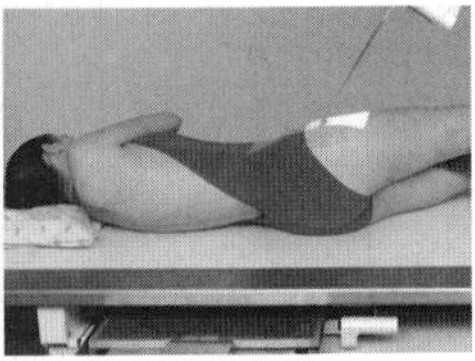

Fig. 9-47 35° LPO axial—CR 30°-45° cephalad.

Position

Supine (AP) or Prone (PA): Patient aligned and centered to centerline
Alternate Oblique: LPO or RAO: Oblique patient 30°-40°
Central Ray: CR 30°-40° cephalad for AP; 30°-40° caudad for PA

AP:
CR to 2″ (5 cm) inferior to ASIS

PA:
CR to enter at level of ASIS

LPO:
CR 2″ (5 cm) inferior and 2″ (5 cm) medial to right ASIS
SID: 40-44″ (102-113 cm)
Collimation: To area of interest
Respiration: Expose at full expiration.

---

kV Range:	Analog and Digital Systems:
	100-125 kV (Single Contrast)
	90-100 kV (Double Contrast)
	80-90 kV (Water-Soluble Contrast Media)

	cm	kV	mA	Time	mAs	SID	Exposure Indicator
S							
M							
L							

9

Bontrager Textbook, 8th ed, p. 523.

Lateral Decubitus and AP/PA Axial Barium Enema

Evaluation Criteria

Anatomy Demonstrated:

- **Lateral decubitus:** Entire large intestine demonstrated
- **AP/PA axial:** Elongated views of rectosigmoid colon

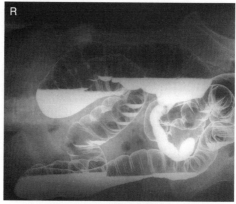

Fig. 9-48 Left lateral decubitus.

Competency Check: _____
Technologist   Date

Position:

- **Lateral decubitus: No rotation** evident by symmetry of pelvis and ribs
- **AP/PA axial:** Less overlap between rectum and sigmoid colon

Exposure:

- Appropriate technique (brightness) to visualize mucosa without overexposing other structures
- Sharp structural margins; no motion

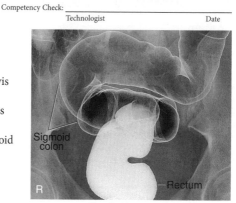

Sigmoid colon

Rectum

Fig. 9-49 AP axial.

Competency Check: _____
Technologist   Date

Abdomen and Common Contrast Media Procedures

9

Intravenous Urogram
AP Scout and Series

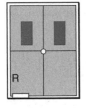

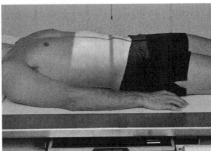

Fig. 9-50 AP IVU.

- 35 × 43 cm L.W. (14 × 17″); 28 × 35 cm (11 × 14″) C.W. for nephrotomography
- Grid
- Include minute marker
- Note that early images may include nephrotomography.
- Shield gonads for males

Position
- Supine, midsagittal plane aligned and centered to centerline, support placed under knees, no rotation

Central Ray: CR ⊥, to center of IR, at level of iliac crest, or 1-2″ (3-5 cm) above crests on long-torso patients with second smaller IR crosswise for bladder area, to include symphysis pubis on lower border of IR

SID: 40-44″ (102-113 cm)

Collimation: To outer margins of IR or area of interest

Respiration: Expose at end of full expiration.

	cm	kV	mA	Time	mAs	SID	Exposure Indicator
S							
M							
L							

kV Range: Analog: 70-75 kV   Digital Systems: 75-80 kV

9

Intravenous Urogram
RPO and LPO

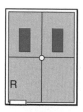

Both R and L posterior oblique projections should be part of routine.

- 35 × 43 cm L.W. (14 × 17″)
- Grid
- Include minute marker
- Shield gonads for males.

Fig. 9-51 30°—RPO.

Position

- Semisupine, 30° oblique to right (or left), flex elevated knee and elbow as shown for support (place angled support under back if needed)
- Align and center abdomen to centerline.
- Center IR to level of iliac crest.

Central Ray: CR ⊥, to center of IR, at level of iliac crest
SID: 40-44″ (102-113 cm)
Collimation: To outer margins of IR or to area of interest
Respiration: Expose at end of full expiration.

	cm	kV	mA	Time	mAs	SID	Exposure Indicator
S							
M							
L							

kV Range: Analog: 70-75 kV   Digital Systems: 75-80 kV

Abdomen and Common Contrast Media Procedures

9

AP and Posterior Oblique IVU

Evaluation Criteria

Anatomy Demonstrated:

- **AP and oblique:** Entire urinary system visualized from renal shadows to symphysis pubis

Position:

- **AP:** No rotation; evident by symmetry of iliac wings; symphysis pubis and top of kidneys included
- **Oblique:** Kidney on elevated side in profile; downside ureter away from spine

Exposure:

- Appropriate technique (brightness) and contrast to visualize kidneys and ureters without overexposing other structures; no motion
- Minute and side markers visible

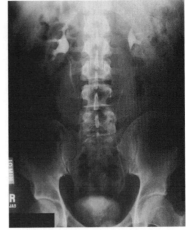

Fig. 9-52 AP—10 minute.

Competency Check: _____
Technologist   Date

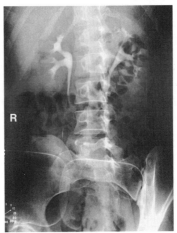

Fig. 9-53 30°—RPO. (From Frank ED, Long BW, Smith BJ: Merrill's atlas of radiographic positioning and procedures, ed 12, St. Louis, 2012, Elsevier.)

Competency Check: _____
Technologist   Date

Intravenous Urogram
AP Erect Postvoid

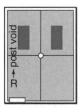

- 35 × 43 cm L.W. (14 × 17″)
- Grid
- Erect and postvoid markers

Position
- Erect, midsagittal plane aligned and centered to centerline, no rotation
- Center IR to iliac crest—ensure that bladder area, including the symphysis pubis, is included at lower IR margin.

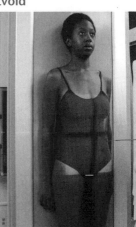

Fig. 9-54 AP erect postvoid.

Central Ray: CR ⊥, to center of IR (at level of iliac crests or ≈1″ or 2.5 cm lower than crest to include bladder area)

SID: 40-44″ (102-113 cm)

Collimation: To outer margins of IR or to area of interest

Respiration: Expose at end of full expiration.

Abdomen and Common Contrast Media Procedures

kV Range:	Analog: 70-75 kV				Digital Systems: 75-80 kV	
	cm	kV	mA	Time	mAs	SID	Exposure Indicator
S							
M							
L							

9

Cystogram—AP

- 30 × 35 cm L.W. (11 × 14")
- Grid

Position

- Supine, midsagittal plane aligned and centered to centerline, legs fully extended
- Center IR to projected CR.

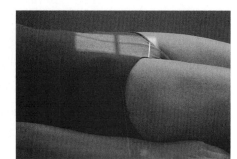

Fig. 9-55 AP—CR 10°-15° caudad.

Central Ray: CR 10°-15° caudad, centered to ≈2" (5 cm) superior to symphysis pubis at MSP (projects pubis inferiorly to better visualize bladder region)

SID: 40-44" (102-113 cm)

Collimation: To outer margins of IR or area of interest

Respiration: Expose at end of full expiration.

	cm	kV	mA	Time	mAs	SID	Exposure Indicator
kV Range:	Analog: 70-75 kV				Digital Systems: 75-80 kV		
S							
M							
L							

9

Bontrager Textbook, 8th ed, p. 559.

Cystogram—Posterior Obliques
(RPO, LPO, and Optional Lateral)

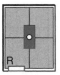

Note: Cystogram routine may not include a lateral because of high gonadal dose.
- 30 × 35 cm L.W. (11 × 14″)
- Grid

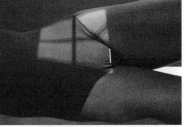

Fig. 9-56 45° RPO.

Position
- Semisupine, 45°-60° oblique (60° oblique best demonstrates posterolateral bladder and UV junction)
- Flex elevated arm and leg to support this position.
- Center patient and IR to CR.

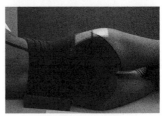

Fig. 9-57 Optional lateral. —CR ⊥, 2″ (5 cm) superior and post to symphysis pubis.

Central Ray: CR ⊥, to ≈2″ (5 cm) superior to symphysis pubis, and 2″ (5 cm) medial to elevated ASIS

SID: 40-44″ (102-113 cm)

Collimation: To margins of IR or area of interest

Respiration: Expose at expiration.

---

kV Range: **AP Oblique**—Analog: 70-75 kV Digital Systems: 75-80 kV
Lateral—Analog and Digital Systems: 80-90 kV

	cm	kV	mA	Time	mAs	SID	Exposure Indicator
S							
M							
L							

AP and Posterior Oblique Cystogram

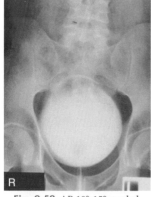

Fig. 9-58 AP 10°-15° caudad.

Competency Check: _____
　　　　　　　　　　Technologist　　Date

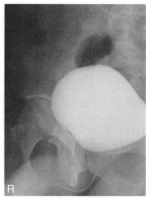

Fig. 9-59 45° posterior oblique.

Competency Check: _____
　　　　　　　　　　Technologist　　Date

Evaluation Criteria

Anatomy Demonstrated:

- **AP:** Distal ureters, bladder, and proximal urethra
- **Oblique:** Distal ureters, bladder, and proximal urethra

Position:

- **AP:** Urinary bladder not superimposed by pubic bones
- **Oblique:** Urinary bladder not superimposed by partially flexed leg

Exposure:

- Appropriate technique (brightness) to visualize urinary bladder without overexposing other structures; no motion

Chapter 10

Mobile (Portables) and Surgical Procedures

Essential Principles for Trauma and Mobile Radiography

The following three principles must be observed for trauma and mobile procedures:

- **Two projections 90° to each other (minimum):** Trauma radiography generally requires two projections taken at 90° (or right angles to each other) while true CR-part-IR alignment is maintained.
- **Entire anatomic structure or trauma area on image receptor:** Trauma radiography mandates that the entire structure being examined should be included on the radiographic image to ensure that no pathologic condition is missed. Additional projections must be taken if the entire structure is not seen on the initial image.
- **Maintain the safety of the patient, health care workers, and the public:** Technologist must maintain the safety and well-being of patients, family/friends, and other health workers during a trauma or mobile radiographic procedure. Safe handling of patients and radiation protection of the patient and others in the immediate vicinity of the exposure is the responsibility of the technologist.

Mobile (Portables) and Surgical Procedures

10

Mobile—AP Chest

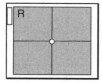

- 35 × 43 cm C.W. or L.W. (14 × 17″)
- Nongrid or grid

Position

- Cover IR with pillowcase or other cover, center to patient with top of IR approximately 2″ (5 cm) above shoulders.
- Elevate head end of bed if possible into seated or semierect position.
- Ensure no rotation of patient.
- If patient is able, rotate shoulders forward.

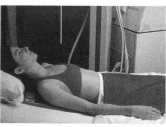

Fig. 10-1 Supine AP chest.

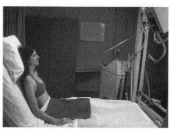

Fig. 10-2 Semierect AP chest.

Central Ray:

- CR 3°-5° caudal from perpendicular to IR so as to be perpendicular to sternum (prevents clavicles from obscuring apices of lungs)
- Center CR to 3-4″ (8-10 cm) below jugular notch.

SID: 48-72″ (123-183 cm). Use greater SID if possible.

Respiration: Expose after second full inspiration.

---

kV Range: Analog and Digital Systems: 90-125 kV*
*Lower kV for nongrid procedures.

Analog:

cm	kV	mA	Time	mAs	SID	IR Size	IR Speed	Grid

Digital:

cm	kV	mA	Time	mAs	SID	IR Size	IR Speed	Grid

Mobile (Portables) and Surgical Procedures

10

310   Bontrager Textbook, 8th edition, p. 577.

Mobile—AP Abdomen (KUB)

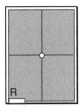

R

- 35 × 43 cm (14 × 17") L.W.
- Grid

Position

- Cover IR with pillowcase or cover.

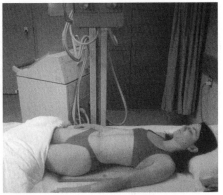

Fig. 10-3 AP supine abdomen.

- Center IR to patient at level of iliac crest.
- Place pads under IR if needed to keep IR level in the soft bed or surface so as to be perpendicular to CR.

Central Ray: CR perpendicular to IR, centered to IR at level of iliac crest

SID: 40-44" (102-113 cm)

Respiration: Expose on expiration

Mobile (Portables) and Surgical Procedures

kV Range:	Analog and Digital Systems: 70-80 kV

Analog:

cm	kV	mA	Time	mAs	SID	IR Size	IR Speed	Grid

Digital:

cm	kV	mA	Time	mAs	SID	IR Size	IR Speed	Grid

10

Mobile—Lateral Decubitus

Abdomen

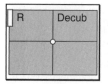

Left lateral best demonstrates free air in right upper abdomen. Must include diaphragm.

- 35 × 43 cm (14 × 17″) L.W. (to anatomy)
- Grid
- Decubitus marker

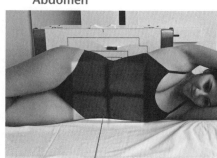

Fig. 10-4 AP left lateral decubitus abdomen.

Position

- Patient turned on left (or right if indicated) side with pads or positioning board under hip and thorax as shown to prevent sinking into soft bed
- Center of IR 2″ (5 cm) above level of iliac crest to include diaphragm
- Ensure no rotation, and that IR is not tilted but is perpendicular to CR.

Central Ray: Horizontal CR to center of IR 1-2″ (3-5 cm) above iliac crest

SID: 40-44″ (102-113 cm)

Respiration: Expose on expiration.

Note: Have patient on side **5 minutes** (minimum) before making exposure; **10 to 20 minutes is preferred.** Ensure that diaphragm and upside of abdomen are included.

kV Range:		Analog and Digital Systems: 70-80 kV

Analog:

cm	kV	mA	Time	mAs	SID	IR Size	IR Speed	Grid

Digital:

cm	kV	mA	Time	mAs	SID	IR Size	IR Speed	Grid

Bontrager Textbook, 8th edition, p. 580.

Mobile (Portables) and Surgical Procedures

10

Mobile—AP Pelvis or Hip

Pelvis

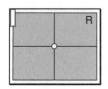

- 35 × 43 cm (14 × 17") C.W.
- Grid

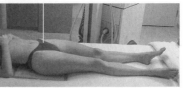

Fig. 10-5 AP pelvis (trauma hip without leg rotation).

Hip Only
- 24 × 30 cm (10 × 12") L.W.
- Grid

Position—Pelvis
- Cover IR with pillowcase or cover, slide IR under patient centered crosswise to patient.
- Top of IR about 1" (2.5 cm) above iliac crest

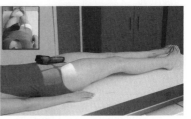

Fig. 10-6 AP hip (with leg rotation).

- Ensure no rotation of patient (equal ASIS distances to IR).
- Internally rotate both legs 15° only if hip fracture is not suspected

Central Ray: CR perpendicular to IR centered to IR and to pelvis or hip

AP Hip: Center CR and IR to hip region (2" or 5 cm medial to ASIS at level of greater trochanter)

SID: 40-44" (102-113 cm)

Respiration: Suspend during exposure.

kV Range:						Analog and Digital Systems: 70-80 kV, Distal Femur 80-90 kV, Proximal Femur/Pelvis		

Analog:

cm	kV	mA	Time	mAs	SID	IR Size	IR Speed	Grid

Digital:

cm	kV	mA	Time	mAs	SID	IR Size	IR Speed	Grid

Mobile (Portables) and Surgical Procedures

10

Mobile—Axiolateral Hip
(Danelius-Miller Method)

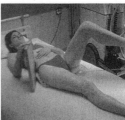

Fig. 10-7 Axiolateral hip.

- 24 × 30 cm (10 × 12″) C.W.
- Grid

Position
- Place folded towels or support under affected hip.
- Place vertical grid against patient's side with top of IR just above iliac crest with face of grid parallel to femoral neck and perpendicular to CR.
- Elevate opposite leg (**Do NOT** support leg/foot on collimator or tube because of risk for burns or electrical shock.)
- Internally rotate affected leg only if unsecured hip fracture is not suspected.

Central Ray: Horizontal CR angled to be perpendicular to IR and femoral neck

SID: 40-44″ (102-113 cm)

Respiration: Suspend during exposure.

kV Range:	Analog: 80 ± 5 kV	Digital Systems: 80-85 kV

Analog:

cm	kV	mA	Time	mAs	SID	IR Size	IR Speed	Grid

Digital:

cm	kV	mA	Time	mAs	SID	IR Size	IR Speed	Grid

10

Bontrager Textbook, 8th edition, p. 590.

Mobile—Modified Axiolateral Hip and Proximal Femur

(Clements-Nakayama Method)

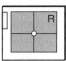

Alternative projection if both limbs have limited movement

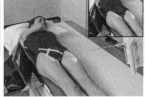

Fig. 10-8 Modified axiolateral projection.

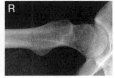

Fig. 10-9 Lateral proximal femur (modified axiolateral projection).

and the inferosuperior projection cannot be obtained
- 24 × 30 cm (10 × 12″) C.W.
- Grid (aligned to CR angle to prevent grid cutoff)

Position
- Patient supine, affected side near edge of table with both legs fully extended
- Provide pillow for head, and place arms across superior chest.
- Maintain leg in neutral (anatomic) position.
- Rest IR on extended Bucky tray, which places the bottom edge of the IR about 2″ (5 cm) below the level of the tabletop.
- Tilt IR approximately 15° from vertical and adjust alignment of IR to ensure that face of IR is **perpendicular** to CR to prevent grid cutoff.
- Center centerline of IR to projected CR.

Central Ray:
- Angle CR **mediolaterally** as needed so that it is **perpendicular to** and **centered to femoral neck** (approximately **15° to 20°** posteriorly from horizontal).

SID: 40-44″ (102-113 cm)

kV Range:	Analog: 80 ± 5 kV	Digital Systems: 80-85 kV

Analog:

cm	kV	mA	Time	mAs	SID	IR Size	IR Speed	Grid

Digital:

cm	kV	mA	Time	mAs	SID	IR Size	IR Speed	Grid

Mobile (Portables) and Surgical Procedures

10

Surgical (Mobile) C-Arm

PA Abdomen (Cholangiogram)

Position and CR

- PA projection (patient supine): Image intensifier on top, tube below

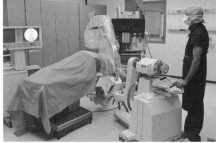

  - Keep intensifier as close to patient as possible to reduce scatter.

- Provide lead aprons or portable shields for all personnel in room.

Fig. 10-10 C-arm being positioned for PA hip or abdomen.

- Maintain sterile field.
- Auto or manual exposure control
- Foot pedal allows hands-free operation by physician of fluoro image as displayed on monitor

Notes:

C-Arm Lateral Hip

Position and CR

- Superoinferior projection
  - Horizontal CR, x-ray tube superior, intensifier inferior
- Ensure sterile field
- Provide lead aprons or shields
- Background exposure field greatest at tube end; operator should stand back away from tube region

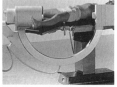

Fig. 10-11 C-arm for lateral hip. *Courtesy Philips Medical System.*

Note: Recommended setup is a reversal of this as an inferosuperior projection because of increased radiation at tube end.

Notes:

Surgical or Mobile Procedures

Procedure Notes:

_____

_____

_____

_____

_____

_____

_____

_____

_____

_____

_____

_____

_____

_____

_____

_____

_____

_____

_____

_____

_____

_____

_____

_____

_____

_____

_____

_____

Mobile (Portables) and Surgical Procedures

10

Appendix A: Reducing Patient Dose

Contributions by W. R. Hedrick, PhD, FACR

There are seven common practices to reduce patient dose during radiographic procedures. They include the following:

- **Minimize repeat radiographs:** A primary cause of repeat radiographs is poor communication between the technologist and the patient. The technologist must clearly explain the procedure to the patient. Carelessness in positioning and selection of erroneous technique factors are common causes of repeats and should be avoided.

- **Correct filtration:** Filtration of the primary x-ray beam reduces exposure to the patient by preferentially absorbing low-energy "unusable" x-rays, which mainly expose the patient's skin and superficial tissue without contributing to image formation.

- **Accurate collimation:** The practice of close collimation to only the area of interest reduces patient dose by reducing the volume of tissue directly irradiated, and the amount of accompanying scattered radiation is decreased.

- **Specific area shielding (gonadal and female breast shielding):** Specific area shielding is essential when radiosensitive organs such as the thyroid gland, breasts, and gonads are in or near the useful beam and the use of such shielding do not interfere with the objectives of the examination. The most common and most important area shielding is gonadal shielding, which significantly lowers the dose to the reproductive organs. Gonadal shields, if placed correctly, reduce the gonadal dose by 50% to 90% if the gonads are in the primary x-ray field.

- **Protection of the fetus:** All women of childbearing age should be screened for the possibility of pregnancy before an x-ray examination.

- **Optimum imaging system speed:** The highest-speed analog (film-screen combination) that results in diagnostically acceptable radiographs is desirable to manage patient dose. Digital imaging systems have essentially replaced film-screen for most radiographic applications. These digital receptors are more sensitive than film-screen and thus have the potential to reduce patient dose.

- **Select projections and exposure factors appropriate for the examination:** Perform projections (pending department approval) that minimize dose to radiosensitive tissues such as the breast and eye. A PA projection will greatly reduce dose to these tissues as compared to an AP projection. Select exposure factors that use highest allowable kV and lowest mAs to further reduce patient dose.

Ethical Practice in Digital Imaging: The wide dynamic range of digital imaging enables an acceptable image to be obtained with a broad range of exposure factors. During the evaluation of the quality of an image, the technologist must ensure that the exposure indicator is within the recommended range. Any attempt to process an image with a different algorithm to correct overexposure is not acceptable; it is vital that patient dose be minimized at the outset and that the ALARA principle be upheld.

To maintain dose at a reasonable, consistent dose level, the following practices are recommended:

- Use protocol-specific kV ranges and mAs values for all procedures.
- Monitor dose by reviewing all images.
- If the exposure indicator for a given procedure is outside of the acceptable range, review all factors, including kV and mAs.

Appendix B: Time-mA (mAs) Chart

Time in Seconds		mA (mAs in Boxes)										
		50	75	100	150	200	250	300	400	500	600	800
1/500	.002	.1	.15	.2	.3	.4	.5	.6	.8	1	1.2	1.6
1/200	.005	.25	.38	.5	.75	1.0	1.25	1.5	2	2.5	3	4
1/120	.008	.4	.6	.8	1.2	1.6	2	2.4	3.2	4	4.8	6.4
1/100	.01	.5	.75	1	1.5	2	2.5	3	4	5	6	8
≈1/80	.013	.65	.98	1.3	1.95	2.6	3.25	3.9	5.2	6.5	7.8	10.4
≈1/60	.016	.8	1.2	1.6	2.4	3.2	4	4.8	6.4	8	9.6	12.8
≈1/50	.019	.95	1.43	1.9	2.85	3.8	4.75	5.7	7.6	9.5	11.4	15.2
1/40	.025	1.25	1.88	2.5	3.75	5	6.25	7.5	10	12.5	15	20
1/30	.033	1.65	2.48	3.3	4.95	6.6	8.25	9.9	13.2	16.5	19.8	26.4
≈1/24	.041	2.05	3.08	4.1	6.15	8.2	10.25	12.3	16.4	20.5	24.6	32.8
1/20	.05	2.5	3.75	5	7.5	10	12.5	15	20	25	30	40
≈1/15	.064	3.2	4.8	6.4	9.6	12.8	16	19.2	25.6	32	38.4	51.2
1/12	.08	4	6	8	12	16	20	24	32	40	48	64
1/10	.1	5	7.5	10	15	20	25	30	40	50	60	80
1/8	.125	6.25	9.38	12.5	18.8	25	31.25	37.5	50	62.5	75	100
1/6	.16	8	12	16	24	32	40	48	64	80	96	128
1/5	.2	10	15	20	30	40	50	60	80	100	120	160
3/10	.3	15	22.5	30	45	60	75	90	120	150	180	240
2/5	.4	20	30	40	60	80	100	120	160	200	240	320
1/2	.5	25	37.5	50	75	100	125	150	200	250	300	400
3/5	.6	30	45	60	90	120	150	180	240	300	360	480
4/5	.8	40	60	80	120	60	200	240	320	400	480	640

Warning: Check tube rating chart for maximum T and mA combinations for larger mAs settings.

New SID	Original SID 36" (91 cm)	40" (102 cm)	42" (107 cm)	44" (112 cm)	48" (123 cm)	60" (153 cm)	72" (183 cm)	100" (256 cm)	120" (307 cm)
30" (76 cm)	.7	.6	.5	.5	.4	.3	.2	.1	.1
36" (92 cm)	1	.8	.7	.7	.6	.4	.3	.1	.1
40" (102 cm)	1.2	1	.9	.8	.7	.4	.3	.2	.1
42" (107 cm)	1.4	1.1	1	.9	.8	.5	.3	.2	.1
44" (112 cm)	1.5	1.2	1.1	1	.8	.5	.4	.2	.1
46" (117 cm)	1.6	1.3	1.2	1.1	.9	.6	.4	.2	.2
48" (123 cm)	1.8	1.4	1.3	1.2	1	.6	.4	.2	.2
50" (128 cm)	1.9	1.6	1.4	1.3	1.1	.7	.5	.3	.2
55" (140 cm)	2.3	1.9	1.7	1.6	1.3	.8	.6	.3	.2
60" (153 cm)	2.8	2.3	2	1.9	1.6	1	.7	.4	.3
72" (183 cm)	4	3.2	2.9	2.7	2.3	1.4	1	.5	.4
100" (256 cm)	7.7	6.3	5.7	5.2	4.3	2.8	1.9	.1	.7
120" (307 cm)	11.1	9	8.2	7.4	6.3	4	2.8	1.4	1

Example 1: Determine mAs with SID changed from 40" to 44". (Look down the 40" column to the 44" box, and locate **1.2** as the conversion factor.) Original mAs = 8.

Answer: 8 × 1.2 = 9.6 or **10 mAs**

Example 2: A chest technique @ 72" is 6 mAs @ 90 kVp. If the SID needs to be decreased to 60", what mAs should be used if other factors remain unchanged?

Answer: Conversion factor is **0.7**. 6 mAs × .7 = **4.2 mAs**

Appendix C: Exposure–Distance Conversion Chart

321

Appendix D: Density–Collimation Field Size Conversions

Accurate collimation of the primary x-ray beam to the area of interest reduces the area and volume of tissue irradiated. This not only reduces patient dose but also improves image quality by reducing the amount of undesirable scatter radiation reaching the image receptor (IR). Therefore reducing the collimation field size reduces the amount of scatter reaching the IR, resulting in less image density. This requires an adjustment in mAs or kV to maintain adequate image density when the collimation field size is significantly reduced.

The **tissue density** and **part thickness,** as well as **screen type and speed,** affect these factors for film-screen systems, but for general purposes the following conversion factors can be used as a suggested starting guide for exposure adjustments.

Field Size–Exposure Conversion Chart (with 400 Speed Screens)

Exposure Field Size Change	Increase in mAs Required	Multiplication Factors
Abdomen 35×43 cm ($14 \times 17''$) $\rightarrow 24 \times 30$ cm ($10 \times 12''$)	25%-35%	1.25-1.35×
35×43 cm ($14 \times 17''$) $\rightarrow 18 \times 24$ cm ($8 \times 10''$)	50%-75%	1.5-1.75×
35×43 cm ($14 \times 17''$) $\rightarrow 10 \times 10$ cm ($4 \times 4''$)	100%-120%	2.0-2.2×
Skull 24×30 cm ($10 \times 12''$) $\rightarrow 8 \times 8$ cm ($3 \times 3''$)	30%-40%	1.3-1.4×

Example: Calculate the new mAs range required for an abdomen when collimation field size is decreased from 35×43 cm ($14'' \times 17''$) to 18×24 cm ($8'' \times 10''$) (collimated gallbladder). Original mAs = 65 @ 80 kV.
Answer: Increase mAs 50%-75%. ($1.5 \times 65 = 98$, $1.75 \times 65 = 114$) New mAs = **98-114.**

Appendix E: Cast Conversion Rule

A cast applied to upper or lower limbs (extremities) requires an increase in exposure. One suggested method for determining exposure compensation is to measure for the increased thickness of the part including the cast and adjust the exposure factors accordingly.

The above method can be used in general, but in addition to the added thickness of the cast, the different densities of cast materials also affect the required exposure adjustments. Therefore the following general cast conversion guide, which makes allowances for both the size and type of cast material, is suggested.

Increase Exposure with Cast

An upper or lower limb with a cast requires an increase in exposure. This increase depends on the thickness and type of cast, as outlined in the following table:

Cast Conversion Chart

Type of Cast	Increase in Exposure*
Small to medium plaster cast	Increase 5-7 kV
Large plaster cast	Increase 8-10 kV
Fiberglass cast	Increase 3-4 kV

*To reduce patient dose, it is recommended to increase kV rather than mAs.
Example: An AP and lateral ankle were taken at 66 kV and 6 mAs demonstrating a fracture. A medium-size plaster cast was applied, and postreduction projections were ordered. What exposure factors should be used?
Answer: **73kV @ 6 mAs** (+7 kV)

Appendix F: Screen Speed Conversion Chart

New Screen Speed	Original Analog Screen Speed											
	25	50	80	100 (PAR)	200	250	300	350	400	500	800	1200
25	1	2	3.2	4	8	10	12	14	16	20	32	48
50	.5	1	1.6	2	4	5	6	7	8	10	16	24
80	.31	.63	1	1.25	2.5	3.13	3.75	4.38	5	6.25	10	15
100 (PAR)	.25	.5	.8	1	2	2.5	3	3.5	**4**	5	8	12
200	.125	.25	.4	.5	1	1.25	1.5	1.75	2	2.5	4	6
250	.1	.2	.32	.4	.8	1	1.2	1.4	1.6	2	3.2	4.8
300	.08	.17	.27	.33	.67	.83	1	1.12	1.33	1.67	2.67	4
350	.07	.14	.23	.29	.57	.71	.85	1	1.14	1.4	2.29	3.4
400	.06	**.13**	.2	**.25**	.5	.63	.75	.88	1	1.25	1.6	3
500	.05	.1	.16	.2	.4	.5	.6	.7	.8	1	1.6	2.4
800	.03	.06	.1	.13	.25	.31	.38	.44	.5	.63	1	1.5
1200	.02	.04	.07	.08	.17	.21	.25	.29	.33	.42	.67	1

This conversion chart allows for a quick approximate conversion of exposure factors when changing from one known speed screen to another.

Example: If the exposure factors for an AP knee with high-speed (400) screen is 4 mAs @ 70 kV, and a 100-speed detail screen is to be used, how much of an increase in mAs is required?

Answer: Find the conversion factor by looking down the 400-speed column to the 100-speed row and locate the conversion factor of **4**. 4 mAs × 4 = **16 mAs.**

To check your answer, convert back from the 100 to the 400 screen technique by looking down the 100 column to the 400 row, for a conversion factor of **.25**. 16 mAs × .25 = **4 mAs** (original mAs).

Appendix G: Grid Ratio Conversion Chart

		Original Grid Ratio (Original Exposure Factors)					
		Non Grid	InSight Grid	5:1 or 6:1	8:1	12:1	16:1
New Grid Ratio	Recommended kV Range	<60-70	60-90	60-75	70-90	70-25 (95-125)	70-125 (95-125)
Non Grid	<60-70	1	.5	.33	.25	.2 (.17)	.17 (.14)
InSight Grid (4 or 5:1 equivalent)	60-90	2	1	.67	.5	.4	.33
5:1 or 6:1	60-75	3	1.5	1	.75	**.6**	.5
8:1	70-90	4	2	1.33	1	.8	.67
12:1	70-125 (95-125)	5 (6)	2.5	**1.67**	1.25	1	.83
16:1	70-125 (95-125)	6 (7)	3	2	1.5	1.2	1

This conversion chart can be used for general grid conversions based on recommended mid-kV ranges of each grid type.

See preceding page for more specific grid conversion considerations.

To use this chart, determine the correct conversion factor (multiplication number) by looking down the chart to the new grid being used, and multiply by this factor.

Example: If **7 mAs** @ 70 kV is the technique for a shoulder using a 12:1 grid, what mAs should be used with a 5:1 portable grid?

Answer: The conversion factor for converting from 12:1 to 5:1 is **.6.**

7 mAs × .6 = **4.2 mAs** at 70 kV.

To check your answer, convert the other way from a 5:1 to a 12:1 grid. An increase in technique would be needed, and the conversion factor is **1.67.** (4.2 mAs × 1.67 = **7 mAs**, the original technique for the 12:1 grid.)

Appendix H: Initials (Abbreviations), Technical Terms, and Acronyms

Following are the more common initials (abbreviations) and acronyms used in imaging departments today and as used in this pocket handbook and in the 8th edition Bontrager Textbook.

General Positioning/Anatomy Terms

AC joints	Acromioclavicular joints
AP, PA	Anteroposterior, posteroanterior projections
ASIS	Anterior superior iliac spine (pelvis landmark)
DP, PD	Dorsoplantar or plantodorsal
LAO, RAO	Left and right anterior oblique projections
LPO, RPO	Left and right posterior oblique projections
MCP	Midcoronal plane (plane dividing the body into anterior and posterior halves)
MSP	Midsagittal plane (plane dividing the body into right and left halves)
SC joints	Sternoclavicular joints
SI joints	Sacroiliac joints
SMV, VSM	Submentovertex or verticosubmental projections

Abdominal Procedure Terms

BE	Barium enema
CCK	Cholecystokinin (hormone, GB procedure)
CNS	Central nervous system
CSF	Cerebrospinal fluid
CTC	Computed tomography colonoscopy
ERCP	Endoscopic retrograde cholangiopancreatography
GB	Gallbladder
GI, UGI, LGI	Gastrointestinal, upper and lower GI
IVP	Intravenous pyelogram (older term)
IVU	Intravenous urogram (accurate term)
KUB	Kidneys, ureters, bladder (abdomen projection)
NPO	Nil per os (nothing by mouth)
OCG	Oral cholecystogram (oral gallbladder procedure)
PTC	Percutaneous transhepatic cholangiography
RLQ, LLQ	Right and left lower quadrant
RUQ, LUQ	Right and left upper quadrant
SBS	Small bowel series
VC	Virtual colonoscopy

Technical Terms

AEC	Automatic exposure controls
Analog	Film-screen imaging system
CR	Central ray (for positioning centering)
CR	Computed radiography—using image plates (IP)
CT	Computed tomography
C.W.	Crosswise (IR orientation to patient); landscape
DF	Digital fluoroscopy
DR	Digital radiography (cassette-less)
FS	Focal spot (large or small)
HIS	Hospital information system
IP	Image plates (used with CR)
IR	Image receptor (film or digital)
L.W.	Lengthwise (IR orientation to patient); portrait
MRI	Magnetic resonance imaging
OID	Object image receptor distance
PACS	Picture archiving and communications system
PBL	Positive beam limitation (collimation)
PET	Positron emission tomography
PSP	Photostimulable phosphor plate receptor (either cassette or cassette-less)
RIS	Radiography information system
SID	Source image-receptor distance
TT	Tabletop (non-Bucky)

Terms Related to Joints of Limbs (Extremities)

ACL, PCL	Anterior and posterior cruciate ligaments (knee)
CMC	Carpometacarpal (wrist)
DIP	Distal interphalangeal (hand or foot)
IP	Interphalangeal (hand or foot)
LCL, MCL	Lateral and medial collateral ligaments (knee)
MCP	Metacarpophalangeal (hand)
MTP	Metatarsophalangeal (foot)
PIP	Proximal interphalangeal (hand or foot)
TMT	Tarsometatarsal (foot)

Terms Related to Cranium and Facial Bones

AML	Acanthiomeatal line
EAM	External acoustic meatus

GAL	Glabelloalveolar line
GML	Glabellomeatal line
IOML	Infraorbitalmeatal line
IPL	Interpupillary line
LML	Lips-meatal line (modified Waters projection)
MML	Mentomeatal line (Waters projection)
OML	Orbitomeatal line
SOG	Supraorbital groove
TEA	Top of ear attachment
TMJ	Temporomandibular joints